Instructor's Manual
Clinical Competencies in
Occupational Therapy

Cindy A. Kief, COTA/L, AP

Instructor and Advisor
Occupational Therapy Assistant Program
Cincinnati State Technical and Community College
Cincinnati, Ohio

Carol R. Scheerer, MEd, OTR/L

Assistant Professor
Department of Occupational Therapy
Xavier University
Cincinnati, Ohio

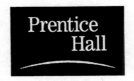

Prentice
Hall

Upper Saddle River, New Jersey 07458

Publisher: Julie Alexander
Acquisitions Editor: Mark Cohen
Editorial Assistant: Melissa Kerian
**Director of Manufacturing
 and Production:** Bruce Johnson
Managing Editor: Patrick Walsh
Production Editor: Publishers' Design
 and Production Services, Inc.
Production Liaison: Cathy O'Connell
Manufacturing Manager: Ilene Sanford
Director of Marketing: Leslie Cavaliere
Marketing Manager: Kristin Walton
Marketing Coordinator: Cindy Frederick
Creative Director: Marianne Frasco
Composition and Interior Design: Publishers'
 Design and Production Services, Inc.
Printing and Binding: Demand Production Center

Prentice-Hall International (UK) Limited, *London*
Prentice-Hall of Australia Pty. Limited, *Sydney*
Prentice-Hall Canada Inc., *Toronto*
Prentice-Hall Hispanoamericana, S.A., *Mexico*
Prentice-Hall of India Private Limited, *New Delhi*
Prentice-Hall of Japan, Inc., *Tokyo*
Prentice-Hall Singapore Pte. Ltd.
Editora Prentice-Hall do Brasil, Ltda., *Rio de Janeiro*

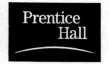

10 9 8 7 6 5 4 3 2 1

ISBN 0-8385-1556-8

Instructor's Manual

CLINICAL COMPETENCIES
in
OCCUPATIONAL THERAPY

Cindy A. Kief • Carol R. Scheerer

Brief Contents

Introduction

Chapter One

EXERCISES 1–17
   a. Study Questions—Key Terms/Readings
   b. Activity—Teaching Strategies
   c. Follow-up

Chapter Two

EXERCISES 18–36
   a. Study Questions—Key Terms/Readings
   b. Activity—Teaching Strategies
   c. Follow-up

Chapter Three

EXERCISES 37–60
   a. Study Questions—Key Terms/Readings
   b. Activity—Teaching Strategies
   c. Follow-up

Chapter Four

EXERCISES 61–75
   a. Study Questions—Key Terms/Readings
   b. Activity—Teaching Strategies
   c. Follow-up

Chapter Five

EXERCISES 76–100
   a. Study Questions—Key Terms/Readings
   b. Activity—Teaching Strategies
   c. Follow-up

Chapter Six

EXERCISES 101–115
    a. Study Questions—Key Terms/Readings
    b. Activity—Teaching Strategies
    c. Follow-up

Appendix

CLINICAL COMPETENCY CHECKLISTS

SECTIONS ONE THROUGH SIX

SELF/PEER GROUP PERFORMANCE EVALUATION

INDIVIDUAL ASSESSMENT OF FEEDBACK

Contents

Introduction   1

Chapter One: Fundamentals 1   3

    Exercise #1: Creating a Vision Statement   3
    Exercise #2: Explaining What We Do   4
    Exercise #3: Prevention and Wellness   5
    Exercise #4: Cultural Awareness   6
    Exercise #5: Learning Your Association's Official Documents   8
    Exercise #6: Ethics in Practice   10
    Exercise #7: Learning the Jargon   12
    Exercise #8: AOTA: Your Professional Organization   15
    Exercise #9: Essential Functions of Occupational Therapy Practitioners   17
    Exercise #10: Frames of Reference   19
    Exercise #11: Occupational Therapy Process   20
    Exercise #12: Practice Guidelines   22
    Exercise #13: Purposeful Occupation   23
    Exercise #14: Occupation: Adaptation   25
    Exercise #15: Occupation: Gradation   27
    Exercise #16: Planning Intervention   28
    Exercise #17: Role Delineation   29

PERFORMANCE SKILLS   30
    Performance Skill #1A   Craft Completion   30
    Performance Skill #1B   Occupational Analysis   30
    Performance Skill #1C   Adapting an Occupation   30
    Performance Skill #1D   Developing Your File   30
    Performance Skill #1E   Cultural Explanation   30

Chapter Two: Fundamentals 2   33

    Exercise #18: Teaching/Learning Process   33
    Exercise #19: Group Observation   35
    Exercise #20: Group Leadership   37
    Exercise #21: Group Treatment   39
    Exercise #22: Managed Care   41
    Exercise #23: Internet   43
    Exercise #24: Clinical Reasoning   45
    Exercise #25: Team Members   47
    Exercise #26: Documentation   48
    Exercise #27: Service Competency   50

Exercise #28: Service Management   51
Exercise #29: Supervision   52
Exercise #30: Professionalism   54
Exercise #31: Public Relations/Service Learning   55
Exercise #32: Advocacy   57
Exercise #33: Research   58
Exercise #34: Licensure   60
Exercise #35: Americans with Disabilities Act   62
Exercise #36: Role Delineation   64

PERFORMANCE SKILLS   66

Performance Skill 2A   Teaching an Occupation   66
Performance Skill 2B   Leading a Group   66
Performance Skill 2C   Public Relations/Service Learning   66
Performance Skill 2D   Therapeutic Use of Self   66
Performance Skill 2E   Mock Interview   66

Chapter Three: Competencies in Pediatric Practice   69

Exercise #37: Observation   69
Exercise #38: The Evaluation Process   71
Exercise #39: Pediatric Intervention Areas   73
Exercise #40: Range of Motion   74
Exercise #41: Positioning and Handling   75
Exercise #42: Reflexes   77
Exercise #43: Play   78
Exercise #44: Feeding   79
Exercise #45: Hand Skills   81
Exercise #46: Handwriting   83
Exercise #47: Activities of Daily Living   85
Exercise #48: Adaptations   86
Exercise #49: Behavior Management   87
Exercise #50: Sensory Integration   89
Exercise #51: School-Based Practice   91
Exercise #52: Early Intervention   93
Exercise #53: Hospital Services and Rehabilitation   95
Exercise #54: Durable Medical Equipment   97
Exercise #55: Vision Loss and Impairment   99
Exercise #56: Hearing Loss and Impairment   101
Exercise #57: Working with Families   103
Exercise #58: Constructing Adaptive Equipment   104
Exercise #59: Intervention Planning   106
Exercise #60: Wellness/Prevention for the Adolescent   107

PERFORMANCE SKILLS   108

Performance Skill 3A   Adding to Your Files   108
Performance Skill 3B   Toy Adaptation   108
Performance Skill 3C   Adaptive Equipment Construction   108
Performance Skill 3D   Standardized Testing   108
Performance Skill 3E   Intervention Planning   109

Chapter Four: Competencies in Psychosocial Practice 111

Exercise #61: Observation Skills 111
Exercise #62: Evaluation of Psychosocial Functioning 113
Exercise #63: Listening and Responding 115
Exercise #64: The Interview Process 117
Exercise #65: Assertiveness 119
Exercise #66: Social Skills 121
Exercise #67: Cognitive Disability 123
Exercise #68: Daily Living Skills 125
Exercise #69: Movement 126
Exercise #70: Leisure Planning 128
Exercise #71: Time Management 130
Exercise #72: Stress Management 132
Exercise #73: Psychosocial Groups 134
Exercise #74: Intervention Planning 135
Exercise #75: Psychological Health, Wellness, and Prevention 137

PERFORMANCE SKILLS 139

Performance Skill 4A   Adding to Your Files 139
Performance Skill 4B   Interview 139
Performance Skill 4C   Planning a Group 139
Performance Skill 4D   Group Activity 139
Performance Skill 4E   Teaching a Basic Life Task 139
Performance Skill 4F   More Practice with Your Teaching 140
Performance Skill 4G   Intervention Planning 140

Chapter Five: Competencies in Adult Physical Rehabilitation Practice 142

Exercise #76: Observation Skills 142
Exercise #77: Standardized Assessment 144
Exercise #78: Muscle Testing 146
Exercise #79: Vital Signs 148
Exercise #80: Sensory Assessment and Reeducation 150
Exercise #81: Transfers and Positioning 152
Exercise #82: Range of Motion 154
Exercise #83: Activities of Daily Living 156
Exercise #84: Wheelchairs 158
Exercise #85: Cognitive Impairments 160
Exercise #86: Perceptual Impairments 162
Exercise #87: Neurodevelopmental Treatment 164
Exercise #88: Proprioceptive Neuromuscular Facilitation 166
Exercise #89: Spinal Cord Injury 168
Exercise #90: Home Management 170
Exercise #91: Assistive Technologies 172
Exercise #92: Therapeutic Adaptations 174
Exercise #93: Medical Equipment in Client Care 176
Exercise #94: Home Health 177
Exercise #95: Work Hardening 179
Exercise #96: Pain Management 181
Exercise #97: Splinting 182

Exercise #98: Upper Extremity Amputations and Prosthetics   184
Exercise #99: Hand Therapy and Physical Agent Modalities   185
Exercise #100: Intervention Planning   187

PERFORMANCE SKILLS   188

Performance Skill 5A   Disability Simulation   188
Performance Skill 5B   Fabrication of Adaptive Device   188
Performance Skill 5C   Adding to Your Files   188
Performance Skill 5D   Activity Adaptation   188
Performance Skill 5E   Intervention Planning   188
Performance Skill 5F   Nontraditional Interventions   188

Chapter Six: Competencies in Geriatric Practice   192

Exercise #101: Getting in Touch   192
Exercise #102: Evaluation in Geriatrics   194
Exercise #103: Safety and Fall Prevention   196
Exercise #104: Adapting Occupation and Environment   198
Exercise #105: Joint Protection, Energy conservation, and Work
   Simplification   200
Exercise #106: Joint Replacement   202
Exercise #107: Remotivation and Reality Orientation   203
Exercise #108: Dementia   205
Exercise #109: Sensory Stimulation   207
Exercise #110: Eating, Feeding, and Dysphagia   209
Exercise #111: Leisure Time   211
Exercise #112: Intervention Planning   213
Exercise #113: Reminiscence and Life Review   215
Exercise #114: Terminal Illness   217
Exercise #115: Activity Programming   219

PERFORMANCE SKILLS   221

Performance Skill 6A   Adding to Your Files   221
Performance Skill 6B   Present a Reminiscing Activity   221
Performance Skill 6C   Prepare/Present Group   221
Performance Skill 6D   Health and Wellness Presentation   221
Performance Skill 6E   Intervention Planning   221
Performance Skill 6F   Home Assessment   222

Appendix   225

CLINICAL COMPETENCY CHECKLISTS   225

Introduction

This book is the instructor's manual (IM) for *Clinical Competencies in Occupational Therapy* (CCOT). It has been written for instructors in accredited occupational therapy and occupational therapy assistant programs or fieldwork educators (practice settings). While it is up to the reader to determine how the content herein best fits into a curriculum, guidelines and suggestions follow.

The content of *Clinical Competencies for Occupational Therapy* (CCOT) is designed to be used in an interactive format. This manual will assist you in utilizing that interactive format. To complete the study questions and activities outlined in the companion book, it will provide you with supplemental information related to study questions and key terms/readings, activity listings and suggested teaching strategies, and follow-up sources for evaluation.

For each exercise you will see first a chart that will help you locate the answers to the correspondingly numbered study questions. Each reference listed is done so by the first author's last name or an abbreviated title of the source. The accompanying key terms will guide you to the specific wording used in the suggested reading so that you can locate the answer easily. In the suggested reading column, the word "index" indicates that the answer can be found by looking up the key terms listed in the *index* of that particular reference. The designation "T.O.C." indicates that the answer can be found when looking up the key terms listed in the *table of contents* of the reference. The word "other" indicates that the answer can be found by looking up the key terms elsewhere and usually appears for documents that have no index or table of contents. Note also that, on occasion, an answer to a study question is not necessarily found in any of the resources, but rather that the students must generate their own ideas for the answer. Such questions are denoted by the word "reflective" in the key term column of the chart. As you go through the process of finding the answers to the study questions, you will become familiar with the content so that you will be prepared to discuss and teach the content to your students.

It is important to note that the references to which you are directed are by no means the only sources from which the answers can be obtained. The chart simply directs you to a complete and thorough answer. You will want to explain to your students that there are often many right answers to such study questions and that each author or reference may give a slightly different view or perspective on the same topic. To the beginning student this diversity can be frustrating; to the advanced student, it can be liberating.

It will facilitate greater understanding of the content and a more interactive discussion if your students answer the study questions prior to your discussion with them. Initially, you may want to allocate class time for answering the study questions, encouraging students to see who can find the answer the quickest. This person or persons may then share his or her technique with the rest of the class to facilitate the learning process of all. By evaluating the thoroughness, timeliness, and accuracy of the answers, you can utilize the study questions to obtain part of the course grade.

Study questions may be assigned according to the specific needs and circumstances of your students. If certain suggested reading resources are not available, some study questions can be deleted, changed, or adapted to fit the materials or readings that are readily available. Additionally, for the occupational therapy assistant (OTA) student, some of the questions on evaluation and frames of reference may need to be omitted or modified.

The second segment of each exercise in this instructor's guide will give you helpful teaching strategies for each activity. The umbers in this section correspond with the numbered activities for the exercises in the CCOT text. In some instances, directions are given to complete the information given in the text. In others, the strategies take the form of ideas regarding methods or formats you might use additionally or alternatively in the teaching process. The strategies are intended as suggestions and tips. When given several options, select the one that most closely fits your need, use all of them, or use the ideas as a springboard to generate your own. The exercises you decide are appropriate can be turned in and used as part of the student's grade.

Finally, the follow-up chart directs you to the appropriate evaluative sources most helpful in assuring that students have integrated the content from the activity. The "Application of Competencies" material located at the end of each chapter of CCOT directs students to determine the most important content of the exercise. It can serve as a review source for students preparing for the national certification examination and as a way for you to determine whether the most salient points have been retained. Documentation of completion of the "Performance Skills" also at the end of each chapter, would be an appropriate addition to a student's portfolio. These skills are evidence of a student's ability to integrate the course content. As an instructor you may want to grade these activities and include the grade as part of a student's final course grade. The checklists in "Appendix B: Self-Awareness", located in the back of CCOT, can be completed at any time in the learning process and would also work well as a portfolio inclusion. This checklist provides the student with a quick, yet thorough way of engaging in the self-reflection process, a tool conducive to learning.

Finally, the "Clinical Competency Checklists," located in the Appendix of this manual are provided for consideration as an inclusion in a student's portfolio. They provide feedback to a student on his/her performance skills as well as the professional behavior expected and needed for administration of effective client care.

It is assumed you will ensure the safety of your students while participating in all of the activities suggested in this manual and the accompanying CCOT. This includes the routine adherence to universal precautions. Students will look to you to model the behaviors you are expected to display.

Assuredly the profession of occupational therapy is changing even as this resource is being written. The academic discipline of occupational science will continue to influence and direct the academic profession of occupational therapy (Zemke and Clark, 1996). By giving you the key terms and location of the answers to the study questions, it is anticipated that you will be able to find the same information in new editions of the references by the same author or new resources by different authors. It will be a challenge for you as an educator to keep up with the changes in the field. It will likewise continually be a challenge for you, as an instructor, to pass along the values, skills, and knowledge needed by future occupational therapy practitioners. It is hoped you will find this instructor's guide and its companion volume to be valuable resources in doing so.

Reference

Zemke, R., and F. Clark (1996). *Occupational Science: The Evolving Discipline.* Philadelphia: F. A. Davis.

Creating a Vision Statement

Study Questions–Key Terms/Readings

Use the chart below to find information addressing each study question. Look up the key terms in the sources given in the suggested readings column. Refer to the index, the table of contents (T.O.C.), or other locations as indicated.

Study Questions	Key Terms	Suggested Readings
1.	OT Information and Resources; General Information; About AOTA: Vision Statement; Mission Statement	www.aota.org
2.	Reflective	Vision/mission statement of host institution
3.	Reflective	Vision/mission statement of host program or department
4.	Reflective	Covey—entire book

Activity–Teaching Strategies

1. Have students share their personal vision/mission statements with each other before creating the class vision/mission statement. Discuss similarities and differences of the individual statements and the strength of having a variety of ideas presented. Discuss Covey's (1986) book and how the information contained therein can be incorporated into their vision/mission statements, educational preparation, and future work with clients.

   Have students return to the vision/mission statement they created throughout the tenure of their academic program to make modifications and revisions. Be sure that each student is supplied with a hard copy of the current revisions for personal use, motivation, and reflection.

Follow-up

Refer to the chart below for the appropriate evaluative source most helpful in assuring that your students integrate the information from this exercise.

Application of Competencies (end of chapter 1 in CCOT)	Performance Skills (end of chapter 1 in CCOT)	Appendix (in CCOT)	Clinical Competency Checklist (appendix in IM)
X			

Explaining What We Do

Study Questions–Key Terms/Readings

Use the chart below to find information addressing each study question. Look up the key terms in the sources given in the suggested readings column. Refer to the index, the table of contents (T.O.C.), or other locations as indicated.

Study Questions	Key Terms	Suggested Readings
1.	The Philosophical Base of Occupational Therapy	AOTA(latest edition)–T.O.C.
2.	Consumer Information: What is OT?	www.aota.org
	Defining Occupational Therapy	Reed–T.O.C.
3.	Scope of Occupational Therapy: Domain of Concern	Moyers–T.O.C.
4.	The Psychosocial Core of Occupational Therapy (1997)	AOTA(latest edition)–T.O.C.
5.	Position Papers	AOTA(latest edition)–T.O.C.
6.	Reflective	
7.a.–f.	Introduction to Occupational Therapy	Neidstadt–T.O.C.
8.	The Guide to Occupational Therapy Practice	Moyers–entire document
9.	Principles of Occupations Used for Intervention	Moyers–T.O.C.
10.	Purpose and Use of This Publication	Moyers–T.O.C.
11.	Occupational Science: Occupational Therapy's Legacy for the 21st Century	Neidstadt–T.O.C.

Activity–Teaching Strategies

1.a.–c. Supplement this activity by using any of the case studies at the end of each chapter and discussing how the explanation of occupational therapy (OT) may be different for each individual. Select a pediatric case study and have the students role-play how they would explain OT to the child's parents. Continue the role-play, explaining the need for OT to this child's insurance company. Have students prepare and present displays or activities that include their definition of OT. Use the displays and activities for OT month.

Follow-up

Refer to the chart below for the appropriate evaluative source most helpful in assuring that your students integrate the information from this exercise.

Application of Competencies (end of chapter 1 in CCOT)	Performance Skills (end of chapter 1 in CCOT)	Appendix (in CCOT)	Clinical Competency Checklist (appendix in IM)
X			

Prevention and Wellness

Study Questions–Key Terms/Readings

Use the chart below to find information addressing each study question. Look up the key terms in the sources given in the suggested readings column. Refer to the index, the table of contents (T.O.C.), or other locations as indicated.

Study Questions	Key Terms	Suggested Readings
1.a.–i.	Prevention of Disability and Maintenance of Health	Christiansen–T.O.C.
2.	Healthy People 2000, U.S. Surgeon General's Report	Christiansen–index
3.	Occupational Therapy in the Promotion of Health and the Prevention of Disease and Disability	AOTA(latest edition)–T.O.C.
4.	Healthy America: Practitioners for 2005	Christiansen–index
5.	Prevention and Disability & Maintenance of Health	Christiansen–T.O.C.
6.a.–h.	Prevention and Disability & Maintenance of Health	Christiansen–T.O.C.
7.	Reflective	Booklets and Pamphlets on Wellness

Activity–Teaching Strategies

1. Collect information that students obtain for this study question and put it into a binder made available for use in the library or classroom. Encourage students to add to the collection as they gather materials and to use the collected materials for future reference. Ask students to find at least one website that gives information on their topics. Post the website addresses on the board for everyone's reference. Instruct students to share personal accounts of participation in wellness or prevention activities.

2.a.–f. Following this activity, discuss activities in which the entire class could participate in order to maintain their health and wellness while in your educational program. Discuss the possibility of the student club sponsoring guests to come speak to the group on different wellness topics such as meditation, tai chi, biofeedback, aerobics, and so on.

Follow-up

Refer to the chart below for appropriate evaluative source most helpful in assuring that your students integrate the information from this exercise.

Application of Competencies (end of chapter 1 in CCOT)	Performance Skills (end of chapter 1 in CCOT)	Appendix (in CCOT)	Clinical Competency Checklist (appendix in IM)
X			

Cultural Awareness

Study Questions–Key Terms/Readings

Use the chart below to find information addressing each study question. Look up the key terms in the sources given in the suggested readings column. Refer to the index, the table of contents (T.O.C.), or other locations as indicated.

Study Questions	Key Terms	Suggested Readings
1.	Reflective	Spector–entire book
2.	Culture, definition of	Neidstadt–index
3.a.–d.	Culture and Other Forms of Human Diversity in Occupational Therapy	Neidstadt–T.O.C.
4.	Cultural competence; Cultural impact	Davis–index
	Multicultural competence; Culture, in occupational therapy process	Neidstadt–index
5.	High-context culture	Davis–index
	Low-context culture	Davis–index

Activity–Teaching Strategies

1.a.–d Have students share their Personal Cultural Charts with the whole group. Have each student prepare a poster representing themselves and their cultures. Use the posters to discuss their cultures and hang them in the class or lab for future reference. Instruct students to bring one item from home that is representative of their cultures and share the significance of this item with the class. Alternatively, instruct students to bring one item representative of their cultures to class and conceal it from the vision of their classmates. Place the items around the room. Have students walk around the room, look at the items on display, and try to identify the person to whom it belongs. Have students write down the identity of the person and the reason they think it belongs to that student.

2.a.–e. Students will inevitably find themselves belonging to several groups. Direct them to select any one of their preference or ask the students to join one of their identified groups that has the fewest members.

3. Provide resources (books, videos, community contacts) for the students on ways to improve their cultural competence. Encourage students to be cognizant of different cultures throughout their educational experience and to think about how intervention may need to be adapted for each individual from a different culture.

Follow-up

Refer to the chart below for the appropriate evaluative source most helpful in assuring that your students integrate the information from this exercise.

Clinical Competency Checklist (end of chapter 1 in CCOT)	Application of Competencies (end of chapter 1 in CCOT)	Performance Skills (in CCOT)	Appendix (appendix in IM)
X	1E		X

Learning Your Association's Official Documents

Study Questions—Key Terms/Readings

Use the chart below to find information addressing each study question. Look up the key terms in the sources given in the suggested readings column. Refer to the index, the table of contents (T.O.C.), or other locations as indicated.

Study Questions	Key Terms	Suggested Readings
1.a.	Essentials and Guidelines for an Accredited Educational Program for the Occupational Therapist	AOTA(latest edition)—T.O.C.
b.	Essentials and Guidelines for an Accredited Educational Program for the Occupational Therapy Assistant	AOTA(latest edition)—T.O.C.
c.	Uniform terminology	AOTA(latest edition)—index
d.	The Philosophical Base of Occupational Therapy	AOTA(latest edition)—T.O.C.
e.	The Occupational Therapist as Case Manager	AOTA(latest edition)—T.O.C.
2.a.	Occupational Therapy Code of Ethics	AOTA(latest edition)—T.O.C.
b.	Knowledge and Skills for Occupational Practice in the Neonatal Intensive Care Unit	AOTA(latest edition)—T.O.C.
c.	Roles and Functions Papers	AOTA(latest edition)—T.O.C.
d.	Standards of Practice for Occupational Therapy	AOTA(latest edition)—T.O.C.
e.	Roles and Function Paper	AOTA(latest edition)—T.O.C.
f.	Standards of Practice for Occupational Therapy	AOTA(latest edition)—T.O.C.
g.	Occupational Therapy and Hospice	AOTA(latest edition)—T.O.C.
h.	Service Delivery in Occupational Therapy	AOTA(latest edition)—T.O.C.
i.	Fundamental Concepts of Occupational Therapy: Occupation, Purposeful Activity, and Function	AOTA(latest edition)—T.O.C.
j.	Occupational Therapy Code of Ethics	AOTA(latest edition)—T.O.C.
k.	Core Values and Attitudes of Occupational Therapy Practice	AOTA(latest edition)—T.O.C.
l.	Bylaws	AOTA(latest edition)—T.O.C.
m.	Glossary of terms for bylaws	AOTA(latest edition)—T.O.C.
n.	Evaluation, defined, Standards of Practice for Occupational Therapy Therapy	AOTA(latest edition)—index
o.	Research, supervision, Occupational Therapy Roles	AOTA(latest edition)—index

Study Questions	Key Terms	Suggested Readings
p.	Clinical Reasoning Skills, defined, knowledge and skills for Occupational Practice in the Neonatal Intensive Care Unit	AOTA(latest edition)—index
q.	Roles and Functions Paper	AOTA(latest edition)—T.O.C.
r.	Roles and Functions Paper	AOTA(latest edition)—T.O.C.

Activity–Teaching Strategies

1. Instruct students to not only "sell" their section but to also inform their audience of the essential information located in their section. Remind the class that a large part of (OT) intervention is using creativity and so they should practice being as creative as possible for this activity. Vote on the classmate most likely to be a success in Hollywood. For added enjoyment, videotape the commercials to play in one of the student's last classes prior to graduation.

Follow-up

Refer to the chart below for the appropriate evaluative source most helpful in assuring that your students integrate the information from this exercise.

Application of Competencies (end of chapter 1 in CCOT)	Performance Skills (end of chapter 1 in CCOT)	Appendix (in CCOT)	Clinical Competency Checklist (appendix in IM)
X			

Ethics in Practice

Study Questions—Key Terms/Readings

Use the chart below to find information addressing each study question. Look up the key terms in the sources given in the suggested readings column. Refer to the index, the table of contents (T.O.C.), or other locations as indicated.

Study Questions	Key Terms	Suggested Readings
1.a.	Occupational Therapy Code of Ethics	AOTA(latest edition)—T.O.C.
b.	Standards of Practice for Occupational Therapy	AOTA(latest edition)—T.O.C.
2.	Occupational Therapy Code of Ethics	AOTA(latest edition)—T.O.C.
3.a.–j.	Standards of Practice for Occupational Therapy	AOTA(latest edition)—T.O.C.
4.	Enforcement Procedures for Occupational Therapy Code of Ethics	AOTA(latest edition)—T.O.C.
5.	Guidelines to the Occupational Therapy Code of Ethics	AOTA(latest edition)—T.O.C.
6.	Who we are; What we do	www.nbcot.org
7.	What we do	www.nbcot.org
8.	What we do	www.nbcot.org
9.	What we do; Disciplinary action	www.nbcot.org

Activity—Teaching Strategies

While playing the game Name That Tune, the students report the correct answer in identifying the Standards of Practice or Code of Ethics. Discuss the standard/ethic to ensure that the meaning and content are understood. This game may also be played patterned after Charades or Pictionary™. Another way of completing this exercise is to conduct a mock trial by giving a situation in which a practitioner violated the Code of Ethics or Standards of Practice. Appoint a lawyer for each situation, as well as a judge and jury. Insist that the students acting as attorneys cite specific information to argue for or against the practitioner. Discuss with the students what they would do if confronted with this situation in the clinic.

Follow-up

Refer to the chart below for the appropriate evaluative source most helpful in assuring that your students integrate the information from this exercise.

Application of Competencies (end of chapter 1 in CCOT)	Performance Skills (end of chapter 1 in CCOT)	Appendix (in CCOT)	Clinical Competency Checklist (appendix in IM)
X			

Learning the Jargon

Study Questions—Key Terms/Readings

1. Using the suggested readings, here is the paragraph with the jargon removed. The interpretation of the acronym appears in boldface.

Dear OT student:

I hope you get to visit the **occupational therapy** department tomorrow at the hospital. They have a large staff with six **registered occupational therapists** and five **certified occupational therapy assistants**, who are all members of the **American Occupational Therapy Association.** They are also training three **occupational therapy assistant students** and two **occupational therapy students.** Some of the things you will observe will be **range of motion** treatment done with the patients who are seen **twice a day.** They are seen in the mornings for **activities of daily living.** The patients are also assisted with meals unless they are **nothing by mouth** per doctor's orders.

If you are **with** the COTA when he is doing ROM, see whether you can tell whether the **right upper extremity** has the same **flexion** and **extension** as the **left upper extremity.** It will be important for you to see a **physical therapist, registered nurse, medical doctor, speech language pathologist, and respiratory therapist secondary/due to** the team approach used at most facilities. **Without** teamwork the patient will not receive the best care, no matter how many **times** you see the patient.

Some of the patients you will see while visiting include patients with **traumatic brain injury, cerebral vascular accident, total hip replacement, cancer, chronic obstructive pulmonary disease, rheumatoid arthritis, acquired immune deficiency syndrome, spinal cord injury, insulin-dependent diabetes mellitus, multiple sclerosis, muscular dystrophy, cerebral palsy, mental retardation, transient ischemic attack,** and **amyotrophic lateral sclerosis.** You will not be seeing a male pt. **diagnosed** with **premenstrual syndrome!**

Remember to be a really great practitioner and **increase** your knowledge you must study **approximately three times a day less than** that will only **decrease** your chances of success and even make it **questionable** if you will succeed. It certainly doesn't matter if you are **greater than** 25 **years old,** as long as your grades are **within normal limits.**

I hope you don't **complain** too much about homework because there will be a great deal, and we want to **rule out** "whiners." You will most certainly notice a **change** in your balance of occupations, which may at times require you to have **stand by assistance.**

When treatment involves a patient who has had a **cerebral vascular accident** you may need to use some **neurodevelopmental treatment, proprioceptive neuromuscular facilitation,** and screen them with the **Allen Cognitive Level**

Test. For treatment you may use a **Baltimore Therapeutic Equipment** work simulator. Another test to try is the **Motor Free Visual Perceptual Test** and check their **Functional Independence Measure** score also. Make sure you read the **American Journal of Occupational Therapy** for the latest information written by a practitioner who is also a **Fellow of the American Occupational Therapy Association** and a **Roster of Honor.**

The children you work with will normally have an **Individualized Education Program** or an **Individualized Family Service Program,** especially if they have **learning disability, attention deficit hyperactive disorder, attention deficit disorder,** or if they have a low **intelligence quotient.** If a **Sensory Integration and Praxis Test** was completed, it may not tell you whether the child can **put on** or **take off** their shirt.

Agencies you will need to deal with in your profession from time to time include the **Health Care Financing Administration, health maintenance organization, National Institute of Mental Health, World Federation of Occupational Therapists, National Association of Retarded Citizens, Joint Commission on Accreditation of Healthcare Organizations, Commission on Accreditation of Rehabilitation Facilities,** and **National Board for Certification in Occupational Therapy.**

You must document in the **problem-oriented medical record** the results of your **sensory integration treatment,** your **manual muscle testing,** the use of the **continuous passive motion machine,** and any **passive range of motion** you have to do to the **bilateral lower extremities.** Be careful in your documentation because they will grade you on the **fieldwork evaluation.**

The HMO may develop a **diagnosis related group** for your patients to determine their **length of stay.** If you write so much that your **metacarpophalangeals, proximal interphalangeals,** and **distal interphalangeals** get sore, you may need a pencil grip.

If you are working in a psychiatric setting, you may work with an **activity therapist.** You may document progress in the **subjective objective assessment plan** format when discussing results of the **Kohlman Evaluation of Living Skills** or the **Bay Area Functional Performance Evaluation.** Your research may take you to the **Diagnostic Statistical Manual (4th Edition)** to see if your pt. has **postraumatic stress disorder** and whether an **electroconvulsive therapy** is standard **treatment.** If your pt. is an alcoholic, he/she may need to go to **Alcoholics Anonymous,** a group called **Substance Abuse and Mental Illness,** or even **a support group for friends and family of alcoholics.**

Next, make sure you search through the **Cumulative Index to Nursing and Allied Health Literature** for the latest copies of **Occupational Therapy Journal of Research, Occupational Therapy in Mental Health, Occupational Therapy in Health Care, Physical and Occupational Therapy in Geriatrics, Physical and Occupational Therapy in Pediatrics,** and the **Canadian Journal of Occupational Therapy.** It will help in your research.

2. If you need to go to the bathroom it is not good or bad, go fast, and remember, stop and look for boys and girls before you come back.

Activity—Teaching Strategies

1. Use any of the terms from the study questions for use in this game, giving the harder terms a higher value. Use complete sentences if you want to make it more challenging.

2. Make sure the students know that it is not appropriate to use abbreviations and jargon with clients and family members.

3. Sentence one: 34 y/o male s/p ®CVA to be seen bid for ADL.

Sentence two: Max. assist x2 and SBA of another to transfer c̄ walker following THR precautions.

Sentence three: UE strength F- in ®UE and P+ in ©UE, WNL for LE

Sentence four: 89 y/o c̄ dx. of TBI, hx of HTN and IDDM.

Follow-up

Refer to the chart below for the appropriate evaluative source most helpful in assuring that your students integrate the information from this exercise.

Application of Competencies (end of chapter 1 in CCOT)	Performance Skills (end of chapter 1 in CCOT)	Appendix (in CCOT)	Clinical Competency Checklist (appendix in IM)
X			

AOTA: Your Professional Organization

Study Questions–Key Terms/Readings

Use the chart below to find information addressing each study question. Look up the key terms in the sources given in the suggested readings column. Refer to the index, the table of contents (T.O.C.), or other locations as indicated.

Study Questions	Key Terms	Suggested Readings
1.a.–h.	Go to the subject as indicated	www.aota.org
2.	Reflective	American Journal of Occupational Therapy (AJOT) (any) Occupational Therapy Practice (OTP) (any) Advance for Occupational Therapy Practitioners (AOTP) (any)
3.a.–b.	Go to the subject as indicated	www.aota.org
4.a.–g.	Reflective	Attend district meeting

Activity–Teaching Strategies

1. Show a video from AOTA that promotes membership. Invite a guest speaker from your local district OT association to speak to your class. Have this individual talk about the importance of involvement in the local OT organization. Encourage students to attend more than one district meeting and/or a special interest section (SIS) meeting. Give extra credit for a paper describing the experience, or require a class presentation. Invite a representative from your student OT club to talk to the students about membership and leadership opportunities. Find out where your state conference is going to be held and solicit volunteers to investigate and ascertain what opportunities there might be for students to become involved. Invite a student who has attended an AOTA national conference to share this experience with your class. Encourage students to prepare a poster presentation for the annual state or national conference.

2. Take pictures of the posters and send them to AOTA. Challenge several students to write an article for OTP and AOTP that demonstrates their support for AOTA.

Follow-up

Refer to the chart below for the appropriate evaluative source most helpful in assuring that your students integrate the information from this exercise.

Application of Competencies (end of chapter 1 in CCOT)	Performance Skills (end of chapter 1 in CCOT)	Appendix (in CCOT)	Clinical Competency Checklist (appendix in IM)
X			

Essential Functions of Occupational Therapy Practitioners

Study Questions–Key Terms/Readings

Use the chart below to find information addressing each study question. Look up the key terms in the sources given in the suggested readings column. Refer to the index, the table of contents (T.O.C.), or other locations as indicated.

Study Questions	Key Terms	Suggested Readings
1.	Reflective	Host educational program documents
2.	Reflective	Local facility documents
3.	Reflective	Local facility documents
4.	Reflective	Local facility documents; Host educational program documents
5.	Reflective	
6.	Reflective; OT Student With Disabilities Title I–Employment	Sladyk–T.O.C. ADA of 1990–T.O.C.

Activity–Teaching Strategies

1.a.–f. To keep your records current and to ensure a comprehensive collection of essential functions from area facilities, ask clinical supervisors to bring updated job descriptions with them whenever they come to campus for a meeting or a workshop. Ask students on fieldwork assignments to bring job descriptions back to school. Keep the collection in a binder that is available for students to refer to as needed.

2. Discuss with students possible strategies to improve the identified skills they need to master. For example, students who are in poor physical condition may be encouraged to exercise more regularly, join a health club, or even receive the assistance of a personal trainer to improve their physical stamina. Others experiencing mental health problems may benefit from receiving counseling or assistance of a support group to improve their interpersonal relationships.

Follow-up

Refer to the chart below for the appropriate evaluative source most helpful in assuring that your students integrate the information from this exercise.

Application of Competencies (end of chapter 1 in CCOT)	Performance Skills (end of chapter 1 in CCOT)	Appendix (in CCOT)	Clinical Competency Checklist (appendix in IM)
X			

Frames of Reference

Study Questions–Key Terms/Readings

Use the chart below to find information addressing each study question. Look up the key terms in the sources given in the suggested readings column. Refer to the index, the table of contents (T.O.C.), or other locations as indicated.

Study Questions	Key Terms	Suggested Readings
1.	Frame of reference	Neidstadt–index
2.	Theories, definition of	Neidstadt–index
3.	Theories, function of	Neidstadt–index
4.	Frames of reference	Neidstadt–index
	Group Guidelines from Seven Frames of Reference	Cole–T.O.C.
5.	Extrapolation, Mosey's steps, group theories	Cole–index
6.	Group Guidelines From Seven Frames of Reference	Cole–T.O.C.
7.	Theories That Guide Practice	Neidstadt–T.O.C.

Activity–Teaching Strategies

1.a.–b. To assign frames of reference to your students, select a case study from the back of the chapter and ask each group to select a frame of reference as well as an activity they might use with that client. Have student present the activity and see if the class can decide which frame of reference they have selected. As an alternative, have students write a statement about their frame of reference on identical pieces of paper. Tape the papers face down on the wall in a Jeopardy game-show format. Turn the papers over one at a time, having students pose questions to identify the frame of reference.

2.a.–d. Have past copies of *OT Practice* available for students to use in decorating their posters.

Follow-up

Refer to the chart below for the appropriate evaluative source most helpful in assuring that your students integrate the information from this exercise.

Application of Competencies (end of chapter 1 in CCOT)	Performance Skills (end of chapter 1 in CCOT)	Appendix (in CCOT)	Clinical Competency Checklist (appendix in IM)
X			

Occupational Therapy Process

Study Questions–Key Terms/Readings

Use the chart below to find information addressing each study question. Look up the key terms in the sources given in the suggested readings column. Refer to the index, the table of contents (T.O.C.), or other locations as indicated.

Study Questions	Key Terms	Suggested Readings
1.	Standards of Practice	AOTA(latest edition)–T.O.C.
	Occupational Therapy Process Model	Reed–index
2.	Assessments (instruments)	Neidstadt–index
	Evaluation	Neidstadt–index
	Preface to the Second Edition	Asher–T.O.C.
3.a.–c.	Evaluation	Neidstadt–index
4.a.	Assessments (instruments)	Neidstadt–index
b.	Observation, of occupational performance, in initial evaluation	Neidstadt–index
c.	Interviewing, in initial evaluation	Neidstadt–index
d.	Introduction to Evaluation and Interviewing	Neidstadt–T.O.C.
e.	Standardized assessment, meaning	Hinojosa–index
f.	Standardized assessment, criterion-referenced testing, norm-referenced testing	Hinojosa–index
g.	Criterion-referenced testing, standardized assessment	Hinojosa–index
5.	Reflective	
6.	Narrative, personal	Christiansen–index
7.	Standards of Practice	AOTA(latest edition)–T.O.C.
8.	Standards of Practice	AOTA(latest edition)–T.O.C.

Activity–Teaching Strategies

1.a.–b. Encourage students to depict the role delineation between the certified occupational therapy assistant (OTA) and the registered occupational therapist (OT) in their drawings. Vote on a winning poster and award a small prize. Since humor can be used as an effective teaching modality, award another prize for the most humorous poster.

2. After you have collected the test questions, split the experts up so that there is

an expert from each different area represented in each newly formed group. Have the experts take turns teaching their specialties to the group. At the completion of the teachings, each member of the class should know each step in the OT process. Give the class a quiz with the test questions submitted by the experts. Give any group that has all members receiving a score on the quiz of 100% five extra points on their next exam.

3.a.–g. Invite humor in the simulations by instructing students to portray an episode from an "OT sitcom" where nothing goes right in the OT process.

4. Once the logo is chosen, have it designed, produced, printed, and distributed to the students. If talent in this area is discovered, draw on the same individual(s) to design other logos for your student group.

Follow-up

Refer to the chart below for the appropriate evaluative source most helpful in assuring that your students integrate the information from this exercise.

Application of Competencies (end of chapter 1 in CCOT)	Performance Skills (end of chapter 1 in CCOT)	Appendix (in CCOT)	Clinical Competency Checklist (appendix in IM)
X			

Practice Guidelines

Study Questions–Key Terms/Readings

Use the chart below to find information addressing each study question. Look up the key terms in the sources given in the suggested readings column. Refer to the index, the table of contents (T.O.C.), or other locations as indicated.

Study Questions	Key Terms	Suggested Readings
1.a.–d.	Introduction	Moyers—T.O.C.
2.	Note: answers can be obtained from AOTA's Uniform Terminology, (Latest Edition)	AOTA (Latest edition)—T.O.C.
3.	Classificaton areas	http://www.who.int/icidh/

Activity–Teaching Strategies

1. This may be played as a drawing game instead of acting. Have the class divided into smaller groups and have each group send one person to the board to draw a representation of the term taken from student-made flashcards. The first group to have someone guess the term correctly gets a point.

2.a. Make a transparency copy of the uniform terminology. Place the transparency on the overhead projector as the class identifies the items to highlight. Have the students use the same transparency for all case studies, but use different colored pens or highlighters for each case. Make a poster of the uniform terminology terms and have it laminated so that it can be used to represent case studies in future exercises.

2.b. Use the designated case studies in 2a for the students to role play. Additionally have students use the Guide to OT Practice: Quick Reference (Moyers, 1999) to explain OT to their families.

2.c. Have each student compile a list of his/her local, state, and national legislators. Discuss the use of their lists when advocating for the profession. Emphasize the need to keep their lists updated and current.

Follow-up

Refer to the chart below for the appropriate evaluative source most helpful in assuring that your students integrate the information from this exercise.

Application of Competencies (end of chapter 1 in CCOT)	Performance Skills (end of chapter 1 in CCOT)	Appendix (in CCOT)	Clinical Competency Checklist (appendix in IM)
X			

Purposeful Occupation

Study Questions–Key Terms/Readings

Use the chart below to find information addressing each study question. Look up the key terms in the sources given in the suggested readings column. Refer to the index, the table of contents (T.O.C.), or other locations as indicated.

Study Questions	Key Terms	Suggested Readings
1.	Purposeful activity	AOTA(latest edition)–index
2.	Reflective	
3.	Occupation	AOTA–index
4.a.	Purposeful play, child	Watson–index
b.	Purposeful activity, adolescent	Watson–index
c.	Purposeful activity, adult	Watson–index
d.	Senior, home improvement, purposeful activity	Watson–index
5.	Occupation performance profile, individualizing	Watson–index
6.a.	Role, defined	Watson–index
b.	Task, defined	Watson–index
c.	Activity, defined	Watson–index
7.	Occupational performance profile, analogy of contexts	Watson–index
8.	Activity(ies), evolution of	Breines–index
9.	Activity analysis, defined	Watson–index
	Task analysis, defined	Watson–index
10.	Activity analysis, mastery of	Breines–index
11.	Task Analysis: An Occupational Performance Approach	Watson–T.O.C.
12.a.–b.	Frames of Reference: Implications for the Use of Crafts	Drake–T.O.C.
13.	Reflective	

Activity–Teaching Strategies

1.a.–c. Determine what age groups are represented by the students as well as the individuals for whom questionnaires were completed. Divide the class into small groups, ensuring that there are a variety of ages represented in each. Discuss the different cultural groups represented. List similarities noticed in these groups. Ask the students what they would like to learn about these as well as other cultures. Encourage them to become more culturally inquisitive in gathering knowledge about the customs of others. Discuss how this information needs to be incorporated in treatment.

2.a.–c.   If time constraints are a concern, have students participate in many activities and select only several for which they will complete the Abbreviated Occupational Analysis Form. Add an active participation component for the students by having them engage in an activity requiring movement, such as dancing, tai chi, or aerobics. Having a large variety of activities will encourage greater discussions as the components of uniform terminology are learned. The Abbreviated Occupational Analysis Form can be completed by individual students or as a class.

3.a.–b.   Since a great deal of energy will be expended in completing such a thorough occupational analysis, select an activity that is fairly easy to learn, for example, basket weaving instead of a cross-stitch activity or making Jell-O™ instead of making tacos. Repeat this entire exercise when teaching craft activities to more thoroughly illustrate the component parts of the new activity to students just learning about task analysis.

4.   Have students complete the Occupational Analysis Form independently and then compare their findings with their peers. Discuss the relativity of the rating system.

5.a.–e.   This exercise can be completed even if students have not had much information on different diagnoses, illnesses, or injuries. Explain that this activity is the beginning of their ability to select appropriate treatment activities for clients. As information is obtained in future courses and gathered from additional experiences, their selection of activities will be influenced. Discuss with students the thought processes they used in arriving at their decisions. As ideas for activities are presented, have the class discuss why or why not the selected occupations might be appropriate.

Follow-up

Refer to the chart below for the appropriate evaluative source most helpful in assuring that your students integrate the information from this exercise.

Application of Competencies (end of chapter 1 in CCOT)	Performance Skills (end of chapter 1 in CCOT)	Appendix (in CCOT)	Clinical Competency Checklist (appendix in IM)
X	1B	B: Analysis of Self	X

Occupation: Adaptation

Study Questions—Key Terms/Readings

Use the chart below to find information addressing each study question. Look up the key terms in the sources given in the suggested readings column. Refer to the index, the table of contents (T.O.C.), or other locations as indicated.

Study Questions	Key Terms	Suggested Readings
1.	Adapting, person-task-environment interventions and	Neidstadt—index
	Grading, of treatment tasks	Neidstadt—index
2.a.–c.	Adaptation	Watson—index
3.a.–g.	Person-Task-Environment Instructions: A Decision-Making Guide	Neidstadt—T.O.C.
4.a.	Skill deficits, person-task-environment interventions and, adapting and	Neidstadt—index
b.	Skill deficits, person-task-environment interventions and, altering and	Neidstadt—index
c.	Skill deficits, person-task-environment interventions and, preventing and	Neidstadt—index
d.	Skill deficit, person-task-environment interventions and, creating and	Neidstadt—index
e.	Skill deficit, person-task-environment interventions, establishing and	Neidstadt—index
f.	Habit deficits, person-task-environment interventions and, adapting and	Neidstadt—index
g.	Habit deficits, person-task-environment interventions and, altering and	Neidstadt—index
h.	Habit deficits, person-task-environment interventions and, preventing and	Neidstadt—index
i.	Habit deficits, person-task-environment interventions and, creating and	Neidstadt—index
j.	Habit deficits, person-task-environment interventions and, establishing and	Neidstadt—index
5.	Adaptive equipment	Ryan(a)—glossary
6.a.–i.	Adaptive equipment, design	Ryan(a)—index
7.	Adaptive equipment, design	Ryan(a)—index
8.	Reflective	

Activity—Teaching Strategies

1. Bring in extra supplies in case students forgot or were not thinking very creatively. Items you could bring include sponges, wooden blocks, twist ties, fabric paint, different colored tape, paper towels, sheets, shoelaces, shoe boxes, food containers, plastic shelving material, contact paper, scraps of wood, and magnets. Get the creative juices flowing by encouraging the most unusual, yet practical ideas. Vote on "most likely to make it big with an invention."

2. Have the students refer to occupational therapy terminology to assist in ideas. Have a note-taker write down all the ideas. When the activity is completed, take the ideas and decide which component or context is being adapted. For any component that was not adapted, try to find a way to adapt it.

3. Do this activity with a particular case study and choose several tasks that may need to be adapted for the individual to be successful.

4. Students may join a small group once craft or activity is completed to share ideas for adaptation. Offer a prize for the student who comes up with the most adaptation ideas. Discourage students from using the same adaptation idea over and over, such as hand-over-hand assist or performing that step for the client.

Follow-up

Refer to the chart below for the appropriate evaluative source most helpful in assuring that your students integrate the information from this exercise.

Application of Competencies (end of chapter 1 in CCOT)	Performance Skills (end of chapter 1 in CCOT)	Appendix (in CCOT)	Clinical Competency Checklist (appendix in IM)
X	1C	B: Analysis of Self	X

Occupation: Gradation

Study Questions–Key Terms/Readings

Use the chart below to find information addressing each study question. Look up the key terms in the sources given in the suggested readings column. Refer to the index, the table of contents (T.O.C.), or other locations as indicated.

Study Questions	Key Terms	Suggested Readings
1.	Grading of treatment tasks	Neidstadt—index
2.	Grading of treatment tasks	Neidstadt—index
3.a.–c.	Purposeful Modifications and Adaptations	Watson—T.O.C.
4.	Grading of treatment tasks	Neidstadt—index
5.	Grading of treatment tasks	Neidstadt—index
6.	Reflective	
7.	Grading of treatment tasks	Neidstadt—index

Activity–Teaching Strategies

1. Have students refer to components of occupational therapy terminology to assist in generating ideas of ways that activities may be graded. Award the winner a prize.

2. Discuss with the students how gradation is used in their curriculum to aid in their learning.

3. Have students join a small group once craft or activity is completed and share ideas. Have a prize for the group that is able to give a different gradation for each component of uniform terminology (AOTA, latest edition).

Follow-up

Refer to the chart below for the appropriate evaluative source most helpful in assuring that your students integrate the information from this exercise.

Application of Competencies (end of chapter 1 in CCOT)	Performance Skills (end of chapter 1 in CCOT)	Appendix (in CCOT)	Clinical Competency Checklist (appendix in IM)
X	1B; 1D	B: Analysis of Self	X

Planning Intervention

Study Questions–Key Terms/Readings

Use the chart below to find information addressing each study question. Look up the key terms in the sources given in the suggested readings column. Refer to the index, the table of contents (T.O.C.), or other locations as indicated.

Study Questions	Key Terms	Suggested Readings
1.	Occupational Therapy Process Model	Reed–T.O.C.
2.	Elements of Clinical Documentation	AOTA(latest edition)–T.O.C.
3.	Elements of Clinical Documentation	AOTA(latest edition)–T.O.C.
4.	Elements of Clinical Documentation	AOTA(latest edition)–T.O.C.
5.a.–d.	Documentation	Neidstadt–index
6.	Documentation, guidelines for	Neidstadt–index
7.	Planning and Intervention	Reed–T.O.C.
8.	Planning and Intervention	Reed–T.O.C.

Activity–Teaching Strategies

1.a.–e. Speak with the instructor who is responsible for teaching the students standardized testing and have this class come to do the testing on your students. You may add any tests that are appropriate. Discuss methods for students to improve their abilities in the areas they have identified. Check goals for relevancy accuracy. Assign due dates for each section of this activity.

2.a.–h. Some students may believe they have no skill to teach. Brainstorm with the class the endless opportunities using the ideas suggested as a starting point. Have the students keep a journal of this experience documenting their progress. On completion of this assignment, have the students present their accomplishments to the class. It is not necessary for the students to actually follow through on teaching and learning these activities, but it would be a plus to assist them in learning note writing and updating goals.

Follow-up

Refer to the chart below for the appropriate evaluative source most helpful in assuring that your students integrate the information from this exercise.

Application of Competencies (end of chapter 1 in CCOT)	Performance Skills (end of chapter 1 in CCOT)	Appendix (in CCOT)	Clinical Competency Checklist (appendix in IM)
X	1D	B: Therapeutic Use of Self-Analysis	X

Role Delineation

Study Questions–Key Terms/Readings

Use the chart below to find information addressing each study question. Look up the key terms in the sources given in the suggested readings column. Refer to the index, the table of contents (T.O.C.), or other locations as indicated.

Study Questions	Key Terms	Suggested Readings
1.	Appendix B	Moyers–T.O.C.
2.	Appendix D	Moyers–T.O.C.
3.	Occupational Therapy Roles	AOTA(latest edition)–T.O.C.
4.	Occupational Therapy Roles	AOTA(latest edition)–T.O.C.
5.	Occupational Therapy Roles	AOTA(latest edition)–T.O.C.
6.	COTA Supervision	Ryan(b)–T.O.C.
7.	COTA Supervision	Ryan(b)–T.O.C.
8.	Occupational Therapy Roles	AOTA(latest edition)–T.O.C.
9.	Reflective	
10.a.–d.	Regulations, supervision, relationship to	Ryan(b)–index

Activity–Teaching Strategies

1. Assign students to complete this activity individually or as a class, inviting the class from a neighboring institution of complementary practitioner students. Plan and prepare for some socialization to occur during this time. Engage all students in an icebreaker activity to help put everyone at ease. Offer food and beverages to help guarantee the success of this joint venture. Additionally, find out from the faculty of the neighboring school when the topic of role delineation will be presented to their students. If schedules can be arranged, combine the two "Introduction to OT" classes. If this idea works, consider holding joint sessions for other topics that would be applicable to both the OT and the OTA student, for example, AOTA, OT Ethics, and Standards of Practice. For additional ideas see the resource Education Unit Task Force (1997), COTA and OTR Education Unit, Bethesda, MD: American Occupational Therapy Association.

2. Have students interview their partners to determine their reasons for entering the profession of occupational therapy.

3.a.–b. Incorporate ideas generated by the students into your host institution's program goals. Submit a write-up of this successful experience for publication

---

Role Delineation

in *Advance for OT Practioners* or *OT Practice*. Suggest a joint faculty presentation at the local, state, or national level. Encourage students to be a part of this presentation also. At the least, submit the experience as a poster session.

4. Have the guests discuss any recent changes that may have occurred in role delineation. Videotape the presentation (with permission) and use the tape in years to come if guest speakers are not available. Invite other speakers from different settings in the future making a videotape library as you go. Use the videotapes and have students compare the role delineations that occur in different settings.

Follow-up

Refer to the chart below for the appropriate evaluative source most helpful in assuring that your students integrate the information from this exercise.

Application of Competencies (end of chapter 1 in CCOT)	Performance Skills (end of chapter 1 in CCOT)	Appendix (in CCOT)	Clinical Competency Checklist (appendix in IM)
X			

Section One

Performance Skill 1A   **Craft Completion**

Include only those activities for which students did not have to complete an Occupational Analysis.

Performance Skill 1B   **Occupational Analysis**

You may produce this computer-generated form for the students. Have students type their analysis so they use their computer skills and you have a more legible document to grade. Post this on the Web for ease of student access. Encourage students to submit this via email. Be sure to identify whether the students are responsible for the adaptation and graded sections on each analysis.

Performance Skill 1C   **Adapting an Occupation**

Solicit information from various fieldwork settings regarding activities they may need adapted. Offer these as choices and have the students actually take these to the settings and give to the OT practitioner. Take pictures of the adaptations for the student to use in their portfolios.

Performance Skill 1D   **Developing Your File**

Once completed, have students share their files as well as the resources they found helpful. They should be encouraged to keep this file organized so that they can add activities to it as directed in the proceding chapters.

Performance Skill 1E   **Cultural Explanation**

Handouts students have obtained from their classmates' presentations will be used throughout their educational experience. These cultural files should be brought to class or actually kept in class and used to supply the needed culture/religion information for the different Case Studies.

References

American Occupational Therapy Association. *American Journal of Occupational Therapy.* Bethesda, MD: Author.
American Occupational Therapy Association Web site: *http://www.aota.org.*
American Occupational Therapy Association. *OT Practice.* Bethesda, MD: Author.
American Occupational Therapy Association. latest edition. *Reference Manual of the Official Documents of the American Occupational Therapy Association, Inc.* Bethesda, MD: Author.
Americans with Disabilities Act of 1990. U.S. PL. 101–336. 42 U.S.C. 12101. *Federal Register,* 56:144, 35543–35691.

Asher, I. E. 1996. *Occupational Therapy Assessment Tools: An Annotated Index.* 2d ed. Bethesda, MD: American Occupational Therapy Association.

Breines, E. 1995. *Occupational Therapy Activities: From Clay to Computers.* Philadelphia: F. A. Davis.

Christiansen, C., and Baum. C. 1997. *Occupational Therapy: Enabling Function and Well-Being.* 2d ed. Thorofare, NJ: Slack.

Cole, M. B. 1998. *Group Dynamics in Occupational Therapy: The Theoretical Basis and Practice Application of Group Treatment.* 2d ed. Thorofare, NJ: Slack.

Costello, E. 1994. *Random House American Sign Language Dictionary.* New York: Random House.

Covey, S. 1989. *Seven Habits of Highly Effective People.* New York: Simon and Schuster.

Davis, C. M. 1998. *Patient Practitioner Interaction: An Experiential Manual for Developing the Art of Health Care.* Thorofare, NJ: Slack.

Drake, M. 1992. *Crafts in Therapy and Rehabilitation.* Thorofare, NJ: Slack.

Everly, J. S. 1996. A goal-setting experiential for the classroom. *Educational Special Interest Section Newsletter,* 6(4): 1–2.

Hinojosa, J., and Kramer, P. 1998. *Evaluation: Obtaining and Interpreting Data.* Sterling, VA: World Composition Services.

International Classification of Functioning and Disability (ICIDH-2) web site: www.who.int/icidh/

Jacobs, K. 1999. *Quick Reference Dictionary for Occupational Therapy* 2d ed. Thorofare, NJ: Slack.

Merion Publications. *Advance for Occupational Therapy Practitioners.* King of Prussia, PA: Author.

Mosey, A. D. 1986. *Psychosocial Components of Occupational Therapy.* New York: Raven Press.

Moyers, P. A. 1999. *The guide to occupational therapy practice.* Bethesda, MD: American Occupational Therapy Association.

National Board for Certification of Occupational Therapy Web site: *http://www.nbcot.org.*

Neisadt, M. E., and Crepeau, E. B. 1998. *Willard and Spackman's Occupational Therapy.* 9th ed. Philadelphia: J. B. Lippincott.

Purdue Research Foundation. 1948. *Purdue Pegboard Test.* Bolingbrook, IL: Samons Preston.

Reed, K. L., and Sanderson, S. N. 1999. *Concepts of Occupational Therapy.* 4th ed. Philadelphia: J. B. Lippincott.

Ryan, S. E., ed. 1995a. *The Certified Occupational Therapy Assistant: Principle, Concepts, and Techniques.* 2d ed. Thorofare, NJ: Slack.

Ryan, S. E., ed. 1995b. *Practice Issues in Occupational Therapy: Intraprofessional Team Building.* Thorofare, NJ: Slack.

Slaydk, K. 1997. *OT Student Primer: A guide to College Success.* Thorofare, NJ: Slack.

Smith, V. 1994. *Occupational Therapy: Transition from Classroom to Clinic-Physical Disabilities Fieldwork Applications.* Bethesda, MD: American Occupational Therapy Association.

Spector, R. E. 1996. *Cultural Diversity in Health and Fitness.* Stanford, CT: Appleton and Lange.

University of Minnesota Employment Stabilization Research Institute. 1933. *Minnesota Rate of Manipulation Test.* Bolingbrook, IL: Samons Preston.

Watson, D. 1997. *Task analysis: An Occupational Performance Approach.* Bethesda, MD: American Occupational Therapy Association.

The Teaching/Learning Process

Study Questions–Key Terms/Readings

Use the chart below to find information addressing each study question. Look up the key terms in the sources given in the suggested readings column. Refer to the index, the table of contents (T.O.C.), or other locations as indicated.

Study Questions	Key Terms	Suggested Readings
1.	The Teaching/Learning Process	Ryan(a)–T.O.C.
2.a.–g.	Teaching/learning process, learning, theories of	Ryan(a)–index
3.	Teaching/learning process, conditions affecting learning	Ryan(a)–index
4.	Communication, verbal, presentation of material in	Purtillo–index
5.	Communication, verbal, presentation of material in	Purtillo–index
6.a.–j.	Communication, verbal, presentation of material in	Purtillo–index
7.	Teaching/learning process, learning task, characteristics of	Ryan(a)–index
8.	Teaching/learning process, teaching process	Ryan(a)–index

Activity–Teaching Strategies

1.a.–f. Use this activity to show your students the importance of direct and specific communication. Point out the difference in the end products when communication is allowed to be a two-way process. Display the completed drawings. Save some of the best (or worst) for future discussions about giving directions. For an extra challenge, have a student or students give their directions to a group of students who are not looking. Compare how different the responses may be, even when the same directions are received by different people.

2.a. Take this opportunity to teach the students a craft or task they need to learn such as metal stamping or copper tooling. Any craft or activity will do. At the same time, help them understand the teaching process.

2.b. As an alternative to making a paper airplane, suggest that students make a similar type of paper object such as a boat, hat, or finger fortune predictor.

2.c. Ensure that students work independently and avoid showing their final products. Allow the "teacher" to give only verbal directions to his or her partner. This technique will be very difficult for students whose written directions are poor. Advise students to be patient and take good notes as opportunity will be given to fix the directions and repeat the process.

2.d. Have students revise their teaching plans incorporating notes from the previously completed activity.

2.e. Small groups of three to five people can be used. On completion of this exercise, discuss the skills used in giving as well as receiving both verbal and written directions. Emphasize the importance of continually critiquing your own communication skills. Discuss how a practitioner's communicative intent will need to be aligned with the client's needs.

Follow-up

Refer to the chart below for the appropriate evaluative source most helpful in assuring that your students integrate the information from this exercise.

Application of Competencies (end of chapter 2 in CCOT)	Performance Skills (end of chapter 2 in CCOT)	Appendix (in CCOT)	Clinical Competency Checklist (appendix in IM)
X	2A	B: Therapeutic Use of Self-Analysis	X

Group Observation

Study Questions–Key Terms/Readings

Use the chart below to find information addressing each study question. Look up the key terms in the sources given in the suggested readings column. Refer to the index, the table of contents (T.O.C.), or other locations as indicated.

Study Questions	Key Terms	Suggested Readings
1.	Group, definition of	Howe—index
2.	Curative aspects of group	Howe—index
3.	Understanding Group Dynamics	Cole—T.O.C.
4.	Understanding Group Dynamics	Cole—T.O.C.
5.	Group stages, identification	Cole—index
	Characteristics of Groups	Howe—T.O.C.
6.	Group norms	Cole—index
7.a.–e.	Role of the Leader in the Functional Group	Howe—T.O.C.
8.	Reflective	

Activity–Teaching Strategies

1.a.–b. If this is a newly formed class, make name tags for the members in group #1 to assist the students who are observing. Before beginning this activity, explain to the observers in group #2 how to illustrate a sociogram. Do so without group #1 hearing the directions to avoid biasing their interactions. Instruct each observer to put the names of the members on the sociogram circle in the identical location so their finished products appear similar. For example, have everyone position student number one at the location of one o'clock (as if the circle were a clock) on the circle. As an alternative to making a poster board, have students engage in a similar group project such as writing a theme song, designing a class logo, or writing a class poem.

2.a.–b. Precede this activity with a discussion about the difference between the content and process of a group. Select any activity for group #2 to participate, such as designing and drawing a class logo or writing a theme song. Encourage the observers to move around so that they can hear members interacting. Discuss how this information might be used in a clinic setting.

3.a.–f. Use the accompanying instructions for making squares in preparation for this activity. Then use the following directions to complete the activity: Give each member an envelope containing pieces of cardboard for forming a square. (Each envelope does not contain the correct pieces for a square). The task of each group is to form five squares of equal size. The members must co-operate by sharing and exchanging so that each person ends up with a square; however, members may not speak to each other or signal that they want a piece. They may only give pieces to one another. Have the established rules of this activity available for reference throughout. Monitor the group's adherence to the rules as there is a tendency to become frustrated and "cheat." Use questions 3.b.–f. to have a discussion analyzing aspects of cooperation in solving a group problem and the behaviors that contribute toward group problem solving or obstruct it. Make careful observations yourself so you can contribute to the discussion. (Directions adapted from B. B. Rider and J. S. Rider, 1999, Book of Activity Cards for Mental Health, Kalamazoo, MI: Authors.)

Follow-up

Refer to the chart below for the appropriate evaluative source most helpful in assuring that your students integrate the information from this exercise.

Application of Competencies (end of chapter 2 in CCOT)	Performance Skills (end of chapter 2 in CCOT)	Appendix (in CCOT)	Clinical Competency Checklist (end of chapter 2 in IM)
X		B: Therapeutic Use of Self-Analysis	

Instructions for Making Squares

To prepare a set, cut out five cardboard squares of equal size, approximately six by six inches. Place the squares in a row and mark them as below, penciling the letters: a, b, c, etc., lightly so they can later be erased.

The lines should be drawn so that when cut out, all pieces marked A will be of exactly the same size, all pieces marked C, of the same size, etc. By using multiples of three inches, several combinations will be possible that will enable participants to form one or two squares, but only one combination is possible that will form five squares six by six inches.

After drawing the lines on the six by six inch squares and labeling them with lower case letters, cut each square as marked into smaller pieces to make the parts of the puzzle.

Mark each of five envelopes: A, B, C, D, and E. Distribute the cardboard pieces in the five envelopes as follows: Envelope A has pieces i, h, e; envelope B has a, a, a, e; envelope C has a, j; envelope D has d, f; and envelope E has pieces g, b, f, and c.

__6"__

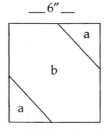 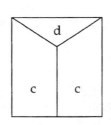 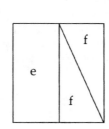 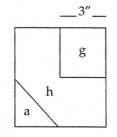

__3"__

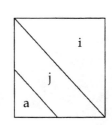

Erase the penciled letter from each piece and write, instead, the appropriate envelope letter, as Envelope A, etc. This will make it easy to return the pieces to the proper envelope for subsequent use when a group has completed the task.

(Used with permission from Rider, B. B. & Rider, J. S. (1999), Book of Activity Cards for Mental Health. Kalamazoo, MI: Authors.)

Group Leadership

Study Questions–Key Terms/Readings

Use the chart below to find information addressing each study question. Look up the key terms in the sources given in the suggested readings column. Refer to the index, the table of contents (T.O.C.), or other locations as indicated.

Study Questions	Key Terms	Suggested Readings
1.	Task roles	Howe—index
	Group roles	Cole—index
2.	Individual roles	Howe—index
	Group roles	Cole—index
3.	Task role	Howe—index
	Group roles	Cole—index
4.	Individual roles	Howe—index
	Group roles	Cole—index
	Patient problems	Cole—index
5.a.–d.	Leadership styles	Cole—index
	Leadership styles, guidelines	Cole—index
6.	Leader, authority, group	Cole—index

Activity–Teaching Strategies

1.a.–b. As a group leader, select a topic that is related to the dynamics of the student class at the time, for example, stress management, time management, peer support, making new friends, performance anxiety, or the like. Use the opportunity to be "therapeutic" with the students so they have the opportunity to see how a group leader performs. On completion, be supportive of any feedback regarding aspects of the group process that you might have done better. Begin this process by critiquing yourself, providing a proactive suggestion for improvement the next time. This experience will give the students an opportunity to experience how feedback should be used in a constructive manner. Emphasize the importance of being open to new ideas.

2.a. Lead several groups with students playing antigroup behaviors so they understand the limit setting that is necessary to lead a cohesive group when antigroup roles are displayed. Alternate the frequency with which antigroup roles are assumed as well as the number of group members. Discuss the effect of same.

2.b. Problem-solve thoroughly about behavior management strategies that may need to be used. Emphasize the hindrance to the therapeutic process when chaos reigns.

Follow-up

Refer to the chart below for the appropriate evaluative source most helpful in assuring that your students integrate the information from this exercise.

Application of Competencies (end of chapter 2 in CCOT)	Performance Skills (end of chapter 2 in CCOT)	Appendix (in CCOT)	Clinical Competency Checklist (appendix in IM)
X		B: Therapeutic Use of Self-Analysis	

Group Treatment

Study Questions–Key Terms/Readings

Use the chart below to find information addressing each study question. Look up the key terms in the sources given in the suggested readings column. Refer to the index, the table of contents (T.O.C.), or other locations as indicated.

Study Questions	Key Terms	Suggested Readings
1.	Activity group, type	Mosey—index
2.a.–g.	Seven-step format	Cole—index
3.	Group Leadership	Cole—T.O.C.
4.	Understanding Group Dynamics	Cole—T.O.C.
5.	Group Guidelines from Seven Frames of Reference	Cole—T.O.C.
6.a.	Group Process	Neidstadt—T.O.C.
b.	Interpersonal learning in groups	Neidstadt—index
c.	Group Process	Neidstadt—T.O.C.
7.	Writing a Group Treatment Protocol	Cole—T.O.C.
8.	Reflective	

Activity–Teaching Strategies

1. For this discussion, review leadership concepts taken from Exercise 20 and from the study questions of this exercise.

2. Observe and assist in critiquing the leader's performance. Assign antigroup roles or allow students to assign the antigroup roles to their peers. Vary the assignments so each leader has opportunity to practice setting limits with a variety of people.

3. Assign specific topics to student leaders that would be of benefit to the entire class, such as assertiveness, time management, stress management, and so on. Ensure that students make copies of any handouts they may need prior to this activity. Use Cole's (1998) Leadership Evaluation form as a guide for providing feedback to the group leader or use another similar evaluation guide of your choice.

Follow-up

Refer to the chart below for the appropriate evaluative source most helpful in assuring that your students integrate the information from this exercise.

Application of Competencies (end of chapter 2 in CCOT)	Performance Skills (end of chapter 2 in CCOT)	Appendix (in CCOT)	Clinical Competency Checklist (appendix in IM)
X	2B	B: Analysis of Self; B: Therapeutic Use of Self-Analysis	X

Managed Care

Study Questions–Key Terms/Readings

Use the chart below to find information addressing each study question. Look up the key terms in the sources given in the suggested readings column. Refer to the index, the table of contents (T.O.C.), or other locations as indicated.

Study Questions	Key Terms	Suggested Readings
1.	A Glossary of Managed Care and Health Insurance Terms; Critical Pathways	AOTA(1996)–T.O.C.
	Answers to crossword puzzle:	
	Across: 1. Critical Pathway 3. PPO 5. Medicaid 7. HCFA 8. DRG 10. Per Diem Rate 12. Gate Keeper	
	Down: 2. Provider 4. Managed Care 6. Medicare 9. HMO 11. Case Management 13. Claim 14. Cost Sharing	
2.	Legislative and Reimbursement Influences on Occupational Therapy: Changing Opportunities	Neidstadt–T.O.C.
3.	Reflective	

Activity–Teaching Strategies

1.a.–e. Discuss with students the need to keep treatment oriented to outcomes that are as functional as possible in every practice setting. Invite a clinician to speak to the students to explain how managed care and the prospective payment system has affected the occupational therapy process.

2. Have students use a case study from their clinical site or the end of the chapter to design an intervention plan incorporating purposeful occupation. Have students share thier ideas with classmates.

3. Acronym abbreviations are as follows: SNF–skilled nursing facility; PPS–prospective payment system; RUGS–reimbursement utilization groups; MDS–minimum data set; CPT–Current Procedures Terminology; ICD-9-Discuss current changes and regulations affecting managed care. Discuss the ethical dilemmas encountered in managed care environments.

Follow-up

Refer to the chart below for the appropriate evaluative source most helpful in assuring that your students integrate the information from this exercise.

Application of Competencies (end of chapter 2 in CCOT)	Performance Skills (end of chapter 2 in CCOT)	Appendix (in CCOT)	Clinical Competency Checklist (appendix in IM)
X			

Internet

Study Questions–Key Terms/Readings

Use the chart below to find information addressing each study question. Look up the key terms in the sources given in the suggested readings column. Refer to the index, the table of contents (T.O.C.), or other locations as indicated.

Study Questions	Key Terms	Suggested Readings
1.a.	Internet, definition	Gibbs—index
b.	Web browser, definition	Gibbs—index
c.	Addresses, definition	Gibbs—index
d.	What Is the World Wide Web?	Pomeroy—T.O.C.
e.	Access provider	Pomeroy—Internet glossary
2.	Surfing the Web for the First Time	Pomeroy—T.O.C.
3.	Internet, literature search via	Reed—index
4.	Internet Resource Directory	Pomeroy—T.O.C.
	Rehabilitation Resources	Pomeroy—T.O.C.
	General Health Care Resources	Gibbs—T.O.C.
	Appendix J: Sample Internet/Software Resources for Person-Task-Environment Transaction Enhancement	Neidstadt—T.O.C.

Activity–Teaching Strategies

1. Compile information gathered by students into a binder, making it available for all students. Emphasize the wide availability of information on the Internet. Caution students to critique the source of the information as there are no regulations concerning the information put on the World Wide Web.

2. Take the students to a computer lab with Internet access at your facility. Have them determine what information can be found on the Internet related to one of the situations described as follows. Make sure students write down each site that led them to the information they needed. Instruct students to use outside sources to supplement the information obtained on the Internet.

   Situation: You have taken a new job at a skilled nursing facility. You need to find out what the current reimbursement guidelines are for Medicare Parts A and B for your clients.

   Situation: You have a client who has multiple sclerosis who would like to return to her job as a factory worker. You need to find out what accommodations she may be eligible for according to the Americans with Disabilities Act (ADA).

Situation: A child that you are treating has been diagnosed with Williams Syndrome. Locate resources that would be helpful to the parents.

3. Discuss with the students how to determine if a website is valid and reliable. Encourage students to bookmark their favorite and most helpful sites. Have students use current issues of *OT Practice* to obtain this journal's periodic suggestions on helpful Internet information. Provide students with a list of your favorite Internet sites to get them started on their search.

Follow-up

Refer to the chart below for the appropriate evaluative source most helpful in assuring that your students integrate the information from this exercise.

Application of Competencies (end of chapter 2 in CCOT)	Performance Skills (end of chapter 2 in CCOT)	Appendix (in CCOT)	Clinical Competency Checklist (appendix in IM)
X			

Clinical Reasoning

Study Questions—Key Terms/Readings

Use the chart below to find information addressing each study question. Look up the key terms in the sources given in the suggested readings column. Refer to the index, the table of contents (T.O.C.), or other locations as indicated.

Study Questions	Key Terms	Suggested Readings
1.	Clinical Reasoning: The Basis of Practice	Neidstadt(1998)—T.O.C.
	Clinical Reasoning	Christiansen—T.O.C.
2.	Tacit knowledge	Mattingly—index
	Clinical Reasoning: The Basis of Practice	Neidstadt(1998)—T.O.C.
3.	Clinical Reasoning: The Basis of Practice	Neidstadt(1998)—T.O.C.
	Metacognition, defined	Christiansen—index
4.a.	Procedural reasoning	Mattingly—index
b.	Interactive reasoning	Mattingly—index
c.	Conditional reasoning	Mattingly—index
d.	Scientific reasoning	Mattingly—index
e.	Narrative reasoning	Neidstadt(1998)—index
f.	Pragmatic reasoning	Neidstadt(1998)—index
g.	Clinical reasoning, facets of, ethical	Neidstadt(1998)—index
5.	Clinical Reasoning	Christiansen—T.O.C.
6.	The Therapist with the Three-Track Mind	Mattingly—T.O.C.
7.	Clinical reasoning, developing expertise in	Neidstadt(1998)—index
8.	Problem solving	Christiansen—index
9.a.–d.	Clinical reasoning, developing expertise in	Neidstadt(1998)—index

Activity—Teaching Strategies

1. Select a "winning" poster(s) to hang in the occupational therapy class or lab area.

2.a.–b. If students have not yet been on fieldwork, give them a situation that you have encountered, one that a clinician has shared with you, or one from a published source. Use the pictures provided by Bride, Twible, and Beltran in *Occupational Therapy: Enabling Function and Well-Being* (Christiansan & Baum, 1997) that illustrate the different reflective framework steps of the clinical reasoning process as visual cues and reminders of the same. Emphasize the importance of being able to verbalize the "tacit" knowledge to which Mattingly (1994) refers. Additionally, have the students solve a clinical situation that you present to them (such as a client with C-6 level of spinal cord injury who will return to the role of mother to two small children) and write down notes on each of the steps. Share the results and discuss the differences.

Follow-up

Refer to the chart below for the appropriate evaluative source most helpful in assuring that your students integrate the information from this exercise.

Application of Competencies (end of chapter 2 in CCOT)	Performance Skills (end of chapter 2 in CCOT)	Appendix (in CCOT)	Clinical Competency Checklist (appendix in IM)
X			

Team Members

Study Questions–Key Terms/Readings

Use the chart below to find information addressing each study question. Look up the key terms in the sources given in the suggested readings column. Refer to the index, the table of contents (T.O.C.), or other locations as indicated.

Study Questions	Key Terms	Suggested Readings
1.	Teams	Neidstadt–index
2.	Teams, interaction models for	Neidstadt–index
3.	Teams	Neidstadt–index
	Reflective	

Activity–Teaching Strategies

1.a.–e. Provide the students with name tags to identify their team role and enable quick identification by fellow team members. Allow students time to review their study question notes and prepare for their roles in the team meeting. Invite a local "team" to present to your class on their various roles and responsibilities. Gather together as many professionals as you can. Discuss the role of team members throughout the students' course of study, emphasizing cooperation and mutual respect as essential to effective client treatment.

2. Emerging practice areas such as ergonomics, driver's evaluation, vision impairment, and violence prevention can be discussed.

Follow-up

Refer to the chart below for the appropriate evaluative source most helpful in assuring that your students integrate the information from this exercise.

Application of Competencies (end of chapter 2 in CCOT)	Performance Skills (end of chapter 2 in CCOT)	Appendix (in CCOT)	Clinical Competency Checklist (appendix in IM)
X			

Documentation

Study Questions—Key Terms/Readings

Use the chart below to find information addressing each study question. Look up the key terms in the sources given in the suggested readings column. Refer to the index, the table of contents (T.O.C.), or other locations as indicated.

Study Questions	Key Terms	Suggested Readings
1.a.–d.	Elements of Clinical Documentation (Revision)	AOTA(latest edition)—T.O.C.
2.	Elements of Clinical Documentation (Revision)	AOTA(latest edition)—T.O.C.
3.	Elements of Clinical documentation (Revision)	AOTA(latest edition)—T.O.C.
4.	Cosignature	AOTA(2000)—T.O.C.
5.a.–j.	Documentation elements, Elements of Clinical Documentation	AOTA(latest edition)—index
6.a.–d.	Documentation, problem-oriented medical record system for	Neidstadt(latest edition)—index
7.	Documentation Review	Acquaviva—T.O.C.
8.	Diagnosis code	Acquaviva—index

Activity–Teaching Strategies

1.a.–c. Have the OT student write the initial progress note including the assessment information and goals for the client. Have the OT student continue the exercise writing a progress note and a discharge summary. Have the OTA student begin this exercise with writing a progress note, which can be generated using the above information, or by using information fictitiously generated. Continue to have the OTA student write a discharge summary. Repeat the process to give students additional opportunity to practice documentation skills.

2. Have students critique their own notes, or collect them as part of a course assignment. Use the information from this checklist as part of a course grade.

3. As the students check each other's work, have them make the corrections they think are needed. Double-check the student's work to ensure accuracy. Have students return the corrected version of each note to the originator. Instruct the student reviewing the notes to comment on the owner's strengths and areas of concern either in writing or verbally.

4. You or a designee will be serving as judge for this activity. You may wish to give information such as a list of everyone's goals, ahead of time to the teams so they can prepare for the trial. Courtroom props can be used to stage or cre-

ate a motivating ambiance. Appoint a sergeant at arms during the proceedings only if necessary!

Follow-up

Refer to the chart below for the appropriate evaluative source most helpful in assuring that your students integrate the information from this exercise.

Application of Competencies (end of chapter 2 in CCOT)	Performance Skills (end of chapter 2 in CCOT)	Appendix (in CCOT)	Clinical Competency Checklist (appendix in IM)
X			

Service Competency

Study Questions–Key Terms/Readings

Use the chart below to find information addressing each study question. Look up the key terms in the sources given in the suggested readings column. Refer to the index, the table of contents (T.O.C.), or other locations as indicated.

Study Questions	Key Terms	Suggested Readings
1.	Service competence, supervision for	Ryan(b)—index
2.	Service competence, supervision for	Ryan(b)—index
3.	Methods to Achieve Competency	Thomson—T.O.C.
4.	Measures to Document Competency; Table 1—Methods of Achieving Competency and the Corresponding Measures of Competency	Thomson—T.O.C.
5.	Supervisor	AOTA(latest edition)—index
6.	Reflective	

Activity–Teaching Strategies

1.a.–c. Select one or more of the magic tricks the students have taught and have them complete an Occupational Analysis (located in Appendix A in CCOT book) on that trick. Discuss how magic can be used in treatment, for example, to improve fine motor coordination or bilateral coordination. Discuss with the students the need to keep accurate documentation regarding their attainment of service competency. Turn to Appendix C in the CCOT book for Service Competency forms that can be used. These may be copied, completed, updated, and placed in the student's portfolio in anticipation of graduation and the attainment of employment as an occupational therapy practitioner.

Follow-up

Refer to the chart below for the appropriate evaluative source most helpful in assuring that your students integrate the information from this exercise.

Application of Competencies (end of chapter 2 in CCOT)	Performance Skills (end of chapter 2 in CCOT)	Appendix (in CCOT)	Clinical Competency Checklist (appendix in IM)
X		C: Service Competency	

Service Management

Study Questions–Key Terms/Readings

Use the chart below to find information addressing each study question. Look up the key terms in the sources given in the suggested readings column. Refer to the index, the table of contents (T.O.C.), or other locations as indicated.

Study Questions	Key Terms		Suggested Readings
1.a.–f.	Management of Occupational Therapy Services		Neidstadt–T.O.C.
2.	Strategic planning		Neidstadt–index
3.	Quality assurance		Neidstadt–index
4.	Service Operations		Ryan(b)–T.O.C.

Activity–Teaching Strategies

1.a.–d. As an alternative to having a guest speaker, assign students to visit or contact by phone various facilities to interview the manager of an occupational therapy department. Send the students out in groups of two or three depending on the number of facilities available. Make arrangements with the appropriate personnel prior to allowing student contact. Have students present the information to the class. Discuss the differences in the various facilities' organizational structures.

2. Obtain an organizational chart from various local facilities, arranging them by practice settings in a binder. Have these charts available for students to use for this exercise.

Follow-up

Refer to the chart below for the appropriate evaluative source most helpful in assuring that your students integrate the information from this exercise.

Application of Competencies (end of chapter 2 in CCOT)	Performance Skills (end of chapter 2 in CCOT)	Appendix (in CCOT)	Clinical Competency Checklist (appendix in IM)
X			

Supervision

Study Questions–Key Terms/Readings

Use the chart below to find information addressing each study question. Look up the key terms in the sources given in the suggested readings column. Refer to the index, the table of contents (T.O.C.), or other locations as indicated.

Study Questions	Key Terms	Suggested Readings
1.a.–d.	Occupational Therapy Roles	AOTA(latest edition)–T.O.C.
	The Function of Student Supervision	AOTA(1991)–T.O.C.
2.	Reflective	
3.	Reflective	
4.	Unit 1: Preparing to Become a Fieldwork Educator	AOTA(1991)–T.O.C.

Activity–Teaching Strategies

1. Make lists of the helpful and not-so-helpful techniques on two different pieces of flip-chart paper. Have the completed lists typed into handouts for the students to keep in their files for future reference, anticipating the role of fieldwork supervisors/educators (practice setting).

2.a.–b. Acquaint students with this information on supervision when needed. Offer the students a workshop on supervision after graduation, using SPICES (AOTA, 1991) information: A more recent version of SPICES is available from AOTA entitled, "Meeting the Fieldwork Challenge: A Self-Paced Clinical Course from AOTA" by S. C. Merrill & P. A. Crist (2000, American Occupational Therapy Association, Bethesda, MD). Use such a workshop for new graduates as a celebration of passing the national certification exam, a class reunion, a means to earn their first professional continuing education units (CEUs), or as a method for training the future generation of fieldwork educators.

3.a.–d. Make sure students get a turn role-playing the supervisor's role to help them empathize with this position. Role-playing done in a small group can be used to ensure empathy will be realized. The use of small groups may also encourage the more reluctant students to take part. Remind the students that they will inevitably be given suggestions for improvement as no "perfect" role-play will be anticipated or achieved.

Refer to the chart below for the appropriate evaluative source most helpful in assuring that your students integrate the information from this exercise.

Application of Competencies (end of chapter 2 in CCOT)	Performance Skills (end of chapter 2 in CCOT)	Appendix (in CCOT)	Clinical Competency Checklist (appendix in IM)
X		B: Therapeutic Use of Self-Analysis	

Professionalism

Study Questions–Key Terms/Readings

Use the chart below to find information addressing each study question. Look up the key terms in the sources given in the suggested readings column. Refer to the index, the table of contents (T.O.C.), or other locations as indicated.

Study Questions	Key Terms	Suggested Readings
1.	Intraprofessional Relationships and Socialization	Ryan(b)—T.O.C.
2.	Occupational Therapy Roles	AOTA(latest edition)—T.O.C.
3.	Personal Life as a Professional	Purtillo—T.O.C.
4.a.–h.	Professional Boundaries	Purtillo—T.O.C.
5.	The Challenge of Creating Professional Closeness	Purtillo—T.O.C.
6.a.–l.	Occupational Therapy Roles	AOTA(latest edition)—T.O.C.
7.	Core Values and Attitudes of Occupational Therapy Practice	AOTA(latest edition)—T.O.C.

Activity–Teaching Strategies

1. Point out the similarities and differences of the various roles. Discuss with students the roles they would like to assume in the future. Have the students complete a time line for their professional development indicating additional education, clinical experiences, and professional roles that they would like to attain.

2.a.–i. Ask students to rate their current status in each area, identifying at least one strategy they want to use to improve their current performance. Survey clinical supervisors at your annual clinical educator's meeting, having them list the professional qualities most important for students to display. Have supervisors depict their perfect students in a drawing. Share these drawings and this information with the students. Invite a clinical supervisor to speak to the students to answer any questions they may have.

Follow-up

Refer to the chart below for the appropriate evaluative source most helpful in assuring that your students integrate the information from this exercise.

Application of Competencies (end of chapter 2 in CCOT)	Performance Skills (end of chapter 2 in CCOT)	Appendix (in CCOT)	Clinical Competency Checklist (appendix in IM)
X			

Public Relations/Service Learning

Study Questions—Key Terms/Readings

Use the chart below to find information addressing each study question. Look up the key terms in the sources given in the suggested readings column. Refer to the index, the table of contents (T.O.C.), or other locations as indicated.

Study Questions	Key Terms	Suggested Readings
1.	Reflective	Local phone book, newspaper, and service agency pamphlets
2.	Reflective	
3.	AOTA Conference	www.aota.org
4.	See home page for promotional topics	www.aota.org

Activity—Teaching Strategies

1. Throughout the year various needs of the community may be brought to your attention. Start a file to keep track of new ideas for service learning projects as well as those projects completed by students in the past.

2. Have students browse current and recent past issues of *OT Week* and *OT Practice* and *Advance for Occupational Therapy Practitioners* for articles and issues pertaining to legislative and reimbursement concerns. *Advance for Occupational Therapy Practitioners* can be accessed online at www.advanceforot.com. Invite the local OT district board member who is the legislative representative to speak to the students about needs in this area.

3. Following the group's discussions, turn to the Performance Skill 2C (located at end of Chapter 2 in CCOT) for directions on how to implement this project. Encourage students to keep accurate records of the activities they complete as a part of this project. Have students take pictures of their "work" for display at a later date. Suggest the presentation of this project as a poster session for the state or national OT conference.

4. Keep a file of past activities performed during OT month to help students get started with ideas. Discuss with them what worked well in the past. AOTA has a variety of resource activities and materials available for this purpose. Students and faculty can work on this project jointly.

Follow-up

Refer to the chart below for the appropriate evaluative source most helpful in assuring that your students integrate the information from this exercise.

Application of Competencies (end of chapter 2 in CCOT)	Performance Skills (end of chapter 2 in CCOT)	Appendix (in CCOT)	Clinical Competency Checklist (appendix in IM)
X	2C		X

Advocacy

Study Questions–Key Terms/Readings

Use the chart below to find information addressing each study question. Look up the key terms in the sources given in the suggested readings column. Refer to the index, the table of contents (T.O.C.), or other locations as indicated.

Study Questions	Key Terms	Suggested Readings
1.	Marketing, planning	Neidstadt—index
2.	Marketing, planning	Neidstadt—index
3.	Marketing, planning	Neidstadt—index
4.	Marketing, planning	Neidstadt—index
5.	Reflective	
6.	Related topics on website	www.aota.org
7.	Reflective	

Activity–Teaching Strategies

1. In addition to the presentation have the students prepare a flier or handout that could be distributed to their target audience. Make copies of the handouts so each student has the information from the other groups for future use.

2. Videotape each group presentation so group members can critique their own performance. Make arrangements with the appropriate community facilities for students to present their information at an agreed upon occasion.

3. Discuss how student's presentations could be used to disseminate information to the list of local, state, and national legislators. Encourage students to write letters make phone calls and visits as a way to inform policy makers of the benefits of occupational therapy practice.

Follow-up

Refer to the chart below for the appropriate evaluative source most helpful in assuring that your students integrate the information from this exercise.

Application of Competencies (end of chapter 2 in CCOT)	Performance Skills (end of chapter 2 in CCOT)	Appendix (in CCOT)	Clinical Competency Checklist (appendix in IM)
X			

Research

Study Questions–Key Terms/Readings

Use the chart below to find information addressing each study question. Look up the key terms in the sources given in the suggested readings column. Refer to the index, the table of contents (T.O.C.), or other locations as indicated.

Study Questions	Key Terms	Suggested Readings
1.	Quantitative research, overview	Bailey—index
2.	Quantitative research, categories of	Bailey—index
3.	Qualitative research, overview	Bailey—index
4.	Qualitative research, strategies	Bailey—index
5.	Data Collection Techniques	Bailey—T.O.C.
6.a.–c.	Occupational Therapy Roles	AOTA(latest edition)—T.O.C.
7.	Introduction	Bailey—T.O.C.
8.	Reviewing the Literature	Bailey—T.O.C.
9.	Occupational Science: Occupational Therapy's Legacy for the 21st Century; Research: Discovering Knowledge through Systematic Investigation	Neidstadt—T.O.C.
10.	Go to AOTF's home page for content listing	www.aotf.org

Activity–Teaching Strategies

1. Alternatively, in "David Letterman" style, have the students prepare a list of the top ten catastrophies that would happen in the field of OT if all research stopped. Select the most humorous and hang this in the class also.

2.a.–f. Have students do this with a partner or in small groups, or by brainstorming with the entire class. Provide ideas to get students started in their thinking. Review a current issue of the *American Journal of Occupational Therapy* or the *Occupational Therapy Journal of Research* or a journal from a related discipline for such ideas. Of the questions generated, select as a group the six favorites.

3. Assign these activities to be completed outside of class time or reserve a computer lab to be used during class time.

4.a.–e. Have students prepare to present their findings orally or in a written format.

5.a.–d. Have students attend a research symposium given by upperclassmen who are further along in their education. Show a videotape of such a presentation if students are not able to attend in person. If you are teaching in an OT school, invite students from the geographically closest OTA program to attend your research symposium. Continue the research process by having OT and OTA students work together collaborating on a research project.

Follow-up

Refer to the chart below for the appropriate evaluative source most helpful in assuring that your students integrate the information from this exercise.

Application of Competencies (end of chapter 2 in CCOT)	Performance Skills (end of chapter 2 in CCOT)	Appendix (in CCOT)	Clinical Competency Checklist (appendix in IM)
X			

Licensure

Study Questions–Key Terms/Readings

Use the chart below to find information addressing each study question. Look up the key terms in the sources given in the suggested readings column. Refer to the index, the table of contents (T.O.C.), or other locations as indicated.

Note: Ohio's Licensure Law (The Laws and Rules Governing the Practice of Occupational Therapy For the State of Ohio, 1998) was used as an example for the chart. Your state license may not address all of these issues. Find the ones that apply.

Study Questions	Key Terms	Suggested Readings
1.	Requirements for License	T.O.C.
	License and Limited Permits	T.O.C.
	Rules to Be Promulgated	T.O.C.
	Denial, suspension, or revocation of license	Rules
	Supervision of limited permit holders and occupational therapy assistants	Rules
	Supervision revocation, or denial of license	Rules
	Fee for escrow of license, restoration	Rules
	Certificate of license, display, copies	Rules
	Continuing education	Rules
	Biennial renewal of license	Rules
	Fee for limited permit	Rules
	Supervision of limited permit holders and occupational therapy assistants	Rules
2.	Occupational Therapy Code of Ethics	AOTA(latest edition)–T.O.C.

Activity–Teaching Strategies

1. If your state does not have licensure, use the registration, certification, or trademark rules and regulations that apply to the practice of occupational therapy practitioners. Construct questions for the game that are true/false, multiple choice, or short answer in nature. Offer a free copy of your state's official current licensure rules to the student(s) who are the winners of this

game.

Follow-up

Refer to the chart below for the appropriate evaluative source most helpful in assuring that your students integrate the information from this exercise.

Application of Competencies (end of chapter 2 in CCOT)	Performance Skills (end of chapter 2 in CCOT)	Appendix (in CCOT)	Clinical Competency Checklist (appendix in IM)
X			

Americans with Disabilities Act

Study Questions–Key Terms/Readings

Use the chart below to find information addressing each study question. Look up the key terms in the sources given in the suggested readings column. Refer to the index, the table of contents (T.O.C.), or other locations as indicated.

Study Questions	Key Terms	Suggested Readings
1.a.–e.	Occupational Therapy and the Americans with Disabilities Act (ADA)	AOTA(latest edition)–T.O.C.
2.a.–d.	Sec. 2 Findings and Purpose	ADA–T.O.C.
3.	Sec. 3 Definitions	ADA–T.O.C.
4.	Sec. 3 Definitions	ADA–T.O.C.
5.	Sec. 101 Definitions	ADA–T.O.C.
6.	Sec. 101 Definitions	ADA–T.O.C.
7.	What Is a Psychiatric Disability Under the ADA	Equal Employment Opportunity Commission–T.O.C.
8.	What Is a Psychiatric Disability Under the ADA	EEOC–T.O.C.
9.	What Is a Psychiatric Disability Under the ADA	EEOC–T.O.C.
10.a.–b.	Disclosure Of Disability	EEOC–T.O.C.
11.a.–f.	Selected Types of Reasonable Accommodation	EEOC–T.O.C.
12.	Direct Threat	EEOC–T.O.C.
13.	Occupational Therapy and the Americans with	AOTA(latest edition)–T.O.C.

Activity–Teaching Strategies

1. In addition to the client problems listed, give the students case studies from the end of any chapter in the CCOT book, along with a vocation and setting where this person was/is working. Have the students list accommodations specific to that client. Assign different case studies with the same job, or the same case studies with different jobs. Invite a guest speaker from a community inclusion program to speak to the students. Similiarly, invite a guest speaker who has a disability and is currently employed, and have that person discuss the accommodations received on the job and in the community. If the students are engaged in paid employment themselves, challenge them to ask their employers what accommodations they would be prepared to make if one of their employees became disabled or if a disabled but otherwise qualified applicant

interviewed for the company. Do they have a plan? Encourage students to share information from this conversation with the class.

Follow-up

Refer to the chart below for the appropriate evaluative source most helpful in assuring that your students integrate the information from this exercise.

Application of Competencies (end of chapter 2 in CCOT)	Performance Skills (end of chapter 2 in CCOT)	Appendix (in CCOT)	Clinical Competency Checklist (appendix in IM)
X			

Role Delineation

Study Questions—Key Terms/Readings

Use the chart below to find information addressing each study question. Look up the key terms in the sources given in the suggested readings column. Refer to the index, the table of contents (T.O.C.), or other locations as indicated.

Study Questions	Key Terms	Suggested Readings
1.	Guide for Supervision of Occupational Therapy Personnel in the Delivery of Occupational Therapy Services	AOTA(2000)—T.O.C.
2.	Guide for Supervision of Occupational Therapy Personnel in the Delivery of Occupational Therapy Services	AOTA(2000)—T.O.C.
3.	Guide for Supervision of Occupational Therapy Personnel in the Delivery of Occupational Therapy Services	AOTA(2000)—T.O.C.
4.	Guide for Supervision of Occupational Therapy Personnel in the Delivery of Occupational Therapy Services	AOTA(2000)—T.O.C.
5.	Service Competency	Neidstadt—index
6.	Supervision Issues when an OT is on Vacation, Leave of Absence, or has Resigned	AOTA(2000)—T.O.C.
7.	Guide for Supervision of Occupational Therapy Personnel in the Delivery of Occupational Therapy Services	AOTA(2000)—T.O.C.
8.	Guide for Supervision of Occupational Therapy Personnel in the Delivery of Occupational Therapy Services	AOTA(2000)—T.O.C.
9.	Occupational Therapy Roles	AOTA(2000)—T.O.C.

Activity—Teaching Strategies

1.a.–e. Divide the standards of practice among the class, giving each group a standard. Instruct the students to take each standard and record what is to be done by the OT, by the OTA, and by both. Share this information with the class so that all will have specific role delineation on each standard. Ask the students what type of supervision is needed if the OTA is functioning at the advanced level of role performance. Ask the students what type of supervision is needed if the practice setting was different.

Add to the topic of role delineation by discussing the use of aides such as activity aide, rehab aide, and OT aide. What would an aide be able to do? Who might supervise the aide? Is an aide licensed in your state? Why would you want to have an aide involved? Why would you not want to have an aide involved? Discuss what is happening in your area regarding the use of aides.

2.a.–j. If this is the first time the students have gotten together in an academic or social setting, engage them in icebreaker activities prior to beginning the activity. Offer refreshments to encourage further interaction. Provide time for the students to become familiar with the instructions and to get their questions answered. Allow students time to discuss with their partners how they will work together on this project. Encourage them to decide how they will proceed. For example, will they meet in person? When? Where? Will they communicate via the phone or postal mail or e-mail? Encourage students to retain all information for this project as well as a summary of their learning experiences as they may wish to share these experiences at a local, state, or national conference. Award students credit towards their grade for successful completion of this project. Discuss the possible use of a project such as this in the clinic when they are supervising OT and OTA students. Present this activity as a good way to have the two levels of practitioners work together. Sands has a chapter in Neidstadt and Crepeau (1998) on the OT/OTA partnership that can be read and discussed. Have small groups of students present different sections of the chapter to their classmates.

Follow-up

Refer to the chart below for the appropriate evaluative source most helpful in assuring that your students integrate the information from this exercise.

Application of Competencies (end of chapter 2 in CCOT)	Performance Skills (end of chapter 2 in CCOT)	Appendix (in CCOT)	Clinical Competency Checklist (appendix in IM)
X	2D, 2E	C: Supervision Log	X

Section Two

Performance Skill 2A

Teaching an Occupation

Have students teach their activity or craft to one other person or to a small group of peers. Give them a specific time frame for completion to guide their choice of activities. As students teach their activity or craft, use the teaching steps as criteria for assigning a grade. Designate how many points each item will be worth.

Performance Skill 2B

Leading a Group

Have a sign-up sheet posted in the room for the students to sign as they decide on the topic for their group activity. This list will ensure that a variety of activities are presented. If there are certain topics you would like covered, have them listed and direct students to sign up for those.

Performance Skill 2C

Public Relations/Service Learning

Have students use this outline to assist them in carrying out their public relations or service learning project. Use any of the following suggestions for projects or generate ideas based on specific community needs: equip a local health clinic with furniture and toys for the children's play area: furnish activities for an apartment building for the elderly; donate toys, food, and health information to a local food pantry; tutor students at a local orphanage.

Performance Skill 2D

Therapeutic Use of Self

Encourage students to solicit feedback from other significant individuals who are, or have been, familiar with their personal and professional qualities, such as family, friends, peers, colleagues, clinical supervisors, instructors, employers, and so on. Have students use the information compiled in the appendix of this IM to get them started. Complete this performance skill as a culminating assignment before graduation. Better yet, have students compose a paper on both entering and exiting the program thus providing an opportunity to have documented evidence of their growth over the time spent in their academic program.

Performance Skill 2E

"Mock" Interview

Contact facilities ahead of time to ask permission for students to call and set up a "mock" interview. Compose a list of occupational therapy directors willing to interview in the area and place each one on an index card. Include the practice setting of the facility, contact person, and phone number on the index card. Have students select a facility based on their interests. To advocate for the profession, have students interview for non-OT but related positions. To obtain interview leads, look in the local newspaper for jobs OTs would be qualified to fulfill, e.g., a local high school is looking for a behavioral consultant. Have students educate the interviewers about the benefits of hiring an occupational therapy practitioner for that position. Have extra facilities/directors available so that if a student is not able to arrange an interview with their first choice (e.g., due to scheduling conflicts), he or she may obtain another card to contact another facility/director. Make a student evaluation for the directors to fill out and return to you. Incorporate this evaluation into the student's grade for the course.

References

Acquaviva, J. D. 1998. *Effective Documentation for Occupational Therapy*. Bethesda, MD: *American Occupational Therapy Association*.

American Occupational Therapy Association. 1991. *S.P.I.C.E.S.: Self Paced Introduction for Clinical Education and Supervision*. Bethesda, MD: Author.

American Occupational Therapy Association. 2000. *COTA Information Packet: 2000* Bethesda, MD: Author.

American Occupational Therapy Association. 1996. *Managed Care: An Occupational Therapy Source Book*. Bethesda, MD: Author.

American Occupational Therapy Association. latest edition. *Reference Manual of the Official Documents of the American Occupational Therapy Association*. Bethesda, MD: Author.

Americans with Disabilities Act of 1990. P.L. 101–336, 42 U.S.C., 12101, Federal Register, vol. 56: 144, 35543–35691.

Bailey, D. M. 1997. *Research for the Health Professional: A Practical Guide*. 2d ed. Philadelphia: F. A. Davis.

Christiansen, C., and C. Baum. 1997. *Occupational Therapy: Enabling Function and Well-Being*. 2nd ed. Thorofare, NJ: Slack.

Cole, M. B. 1998. *Group Dynamics in Occupational Therapy: The Theoretical Basis and Practice Application of Group Treatment*. Thorofare, NJ: Slack.

Equal Employment Opportunity Commission. 1997. *EEOC Enforcement Guidance: The Americans with Disabilities Act and Psychiatric Disabilities*. 915.002.

Gibbs, S., M. Sullivan-Fowler, and N. W. Rowe. 1996. *Mosby's Medical Surfari: A Guide to Exploring the Internet and Discovering the Top Health Care Resources*. Chicago: Mosby.

Howe, M. C., and S. L. Schwartzberg. 1995. *A Functional Approach to Group Work in Occupational Therapy*. Philadelphia: J. B. Lippincott.

Korb, K. L., S. D. Azok, and E. A. Leutenberg. 1989. *Life Management Skills: Reproducible Activity Handouts Created for Facilitators*. Beechwood, OH: Wellness Reproduction.

Korb-Khalsa, K. L., S. D. Azok, and E. A. Leutenberg. 1993. *Life Management Skills II: Reproducible Activity Handouts Created for Facilitators*. Beechwood, OH: Wellness Reproduction.

Korb-Khalsa, K. L., S. D. Azok, and E. A. Leutenberg. 1995a. *Life Management Skills III: Reproducible Activity Handouts Created for Facilitators*. Beechwood, OH: Wellness Reproduction.

Korb-Khalsa, K. L., S. D. Azok, and E. A. Leutenberg. 1995b. *S.E.A.L.S. +Plus*. Beechwood, OH: Wellness Reproduction.

Mattingly, C., and M. H. Fleming. 1994. *Clinical Reasoning: Focus of Inquiry in a Therapeutic Practice*. Philadelphia: F. A. Davis.

Mosey, A. C. 1986. *Psychosocial Components of Occupational Therapy*. New York: Raven Press.

Neidstadt, M. E. 1996. "Teaching Strategies for the Development of Clinical Reasoning." *American Journal of Occupational Therapy*, 50(8): 676–684.

Neidstadt, M. E., and E. B. Crepeau. 1998. *Willard and Spackman's Occupational Therapy*. 9th ed. Philadelphia: J. B. Lippincott.

Pomeroy, B. 1997. *Beginnernet in Rehabilitation: A Beginner's Guide to the Internet—*

the World Wide Web. Thorofare, NJ: Slack.

Purtilo, R., and A. Haddad. 1996. *Health Professional and Patient Interaction.* Philadelphia: W. B. Saunders.

Reed, K. L., and S. N. Sanderson. 1999. *Concepts of Occupational Therapy.* 4th ed. Philadelphia: Lippincott Williams & Wilkins.

Rider, B. B., and J. S. Rider. 1999. *Book of Activity Cards for Mental Health.* Kalamazoo, MI: Authors.

Ryan, S. E., ed. 1995a. *The Certified Occupational Therapy Assistant: Principles, Concepts and Techniques.* 2d ed. Thorofare, NJ: Slack.

Ryan, S. E., ed. 1995b. *Practice Issues in Occupational Therapy: Intraprofessional Team Building.* Thorofare, NJ: Slack.

Thomson, L. K., D. Lieberman, R. Murphy, E. Wendt, J. Poole, and S. D. Hertfelder. 1995. *Developing, Maintaining, and Updating Competency in Occupational Therapy: A Guide to Self-Appraisal.* Bethesda, MD: American Occupational Therapy Association.

EXERCISE **37**

Observation

Study Questions—Key Terms/Readings

Use the chart below to find information addressing each study question. Look up the key terms in the sources given in the suggested readings column. Refer to the index, the table of contents (T.O.C.), or other locations as indicated.

Study Questions	Key Terms	Suggested Readings
1.	Observation, assessment tool for	Dunn—index
2.	Skilled observation	Case-Smith—index
3.	Observation, components of	Dunn—index
4.	Skilled observation	Case-Smith—index
5.	Assessment, clinical guide	Parham—index
6.	Skilled observation	Case-Smith—index
7.	Skilled observation	Case-Smith—index
8.	Assessment, clinical	Parham—index
9.a.–m.	Clinical observation, of neuromotor skills	Case-Smith—index
10.a.–d.	Clinical observation, in sensory integrative dysfunction	Case-Smith—index
11.	Observation, informal, in sensory integrative dysfunction assessment	Case-Smith—index

Activity—Teaching Strategies

1. Obtain permission for your students to observe children at a local day care facility. Keep in mind that some facilities allow students to interact with the children while others allow them to observe on the sidelines or through two-way mirrors. Have students write their notes immediately following the observation. Alternatively, have students complete the assignment at a location other than a day care facility, such as the local YMCA, a community park, or in their own neighborhood.

2. Assist students in writing the clear, accurate, and succinct observations. If two or more students observed the same child, have them work together and generate a revised observation report combining both of their observations. Discuss components of the normal development the students observed. Discuss any atypical behavior observed.

3. Have students complete this activity at their fieldwork site. Alternatively, provide a videotape of a child for them to view. Making a videotape of two children participating in directed activities, one who is typical and one who is receiving therapy services, would allow you to assign either child for students

to observe. A sibling of a child who is receiving intervention may be more than willing to assist in making a "movie." Offer a copy of the videotape to the parents for a keepsake. Once a videotape is made, be sure to save it because parts of the videotape may be used for other purposes throughout your teaching career.

4. Following the student's summary of the skills, provide them with suggestions for improvement. Have students complete observation reports on several additional activities from the videotape. Allow the students to view the videotape in the library, write up their observations, and then check them with yours.

Follow-up

Refer to the chart below for the appropriate evaluative source most helpful in assuring that your students integrate the information from this exercise.

Application of Competencies (end of chapter 3 in CCOT)	Performance Skills (end of chapter 3 in CCOT)	Appendix (in CCOT)	Clinical Competency Checklist (appendix in IM)
X		B: Therapeutic Use of Self Analysis	

The Evaluation Process

Study Questions–Key Terms/Readings

Use the chart below to find information addressing each study question. Look up the key terms in the sources given in the suggested readings column. Refer to the index, the table of contents (T.O.C.), or other locations as indicated.

Study Questions	Key Terms	Suggested Readings
1.	Assessment in pediatric occupational therapy	Case-Smith—index
	Assessment of IADL	Case-Smith—index
	Occupational Therapy Assessment in Pediatrics: Purpose, Process, and Methods of Evaluation	Case-Smith—T.O.C.
	Norm-referenced tests	Case-Smith—index
	Norm-referenced tests	Case-Smith—index
2.	Standardized test	Hinojosa—index
3.	Standardized test	Hinojosa—index
4.	Reliability, defined; Validity, defined	Hinojosa—index
5.	Interrater reliability; Reflective	Hinojosa—index, other
6.	Standardized tests, component use of	Case-Smith—index
7.	Standards of Practice for Occupational Therapy	AOTA(1998)—T.O.C.
8.a.–d.	Calculating the Child's Age & Drawing the Age Line	Frankenburg—T.O.C.
9.	Calculating the Child's Age & Drawing the Age Line	Frankenburg—T.O.C.
10.a.–d.	Administration and Interpretation: Test Administration	Frankenburg—T.O.C.
11.	Administration and Interpretation: Test Administration	Frankenburg—T.O.C.
12.	Administration and Interpretation: Test Administration	Frankenburg—T.O.C.
13.	Administration and Interpretation, Interpretation, Interpretation of Individual Items	Frankenburg—T.O.C.

Activity–Teaching Strategies

1. Have students take turns assuming the role of the OT practitioner and then the role of the parent. Fabricate situations ahead of time to make the interviews more difficult and realistic. Situations may include, but are not limited to, parents who are being forced to participate because of neglect or abuse charges; parents who report living in extremely unfavorable conditions; parents who are extremely anxious that something is terribly wrong with their child; or parents who are deaf and have difficulty communicating. Write these situa-

tions on index cards ahead of time, having students take turns selecting the index card describing the scenario to portray.

2. If class time is not adequate, require students to watch the videotape outside of class time.

3. Have students role-play unusual situations to give them an opportunity to problem solve on their feet; for example, have the parent assume a disability of mild mental retardation.

4. Prior to practicing the administration, ensure that the students are proficient in calculating the child's age. One way to test this proficiency is to have test dates and dates of births on index cards and give one index card to each student. Have them calculate the child's age, draw the age line for that age, and then circle one item in each section where testing will begin. Pass the card to the left and have the students repeat the process until you feel they are competent in these skills. Have the students administer the entire test for one of the ages they have calculated.

   Students need to pass the Denver II proficiency tests before administering the Denver II to a child. Proficiency tests and guidelines can be found in the *Denver II: Technical Manual* by W. K. Frankenburg, J. Dodds, P. Archer, B. Bresnick, P. Maschka, N. Edelman, and H. Shapiro (1996) (available from Denver Developmental Materials, Inc. Denver, CO)

5.a.–b. Prepare a videotaped presentation ahead of time. Make a videotape of you administering the test or obtain a videotape from a clinician who has permission to share this with you. If you have the videotaping technology, the clinician may be more than willing to allow you to tape as long as you give him or her a copy of the tape for future educational purposes.

6. See Asher (1996) for a listing of other assessments appropriate to administer to the pediatric population.

Follow-up

Refer to the chart below for the appropriate evaluative source most helpful in assuring that your students integrate the information from this exercise.

Application of Competencies (end of chapter 3 in CCOT)	Performance Skills (end of chapter 3 in CCOT)	Appendix (in CCOT)	Clinical Competency Checklist (appendix in IM)
X	3D	B: Therapeutic Use of Self-Analysis	X

Pediatric Intervention Areas

Study Questions–Key Terms/Readings

Use the chart below to find information addressing each study question. Look up the key terms in the sources given in the suggested readings column. Refer to the index, the table of contents (T.O.C.), or other locations as indicated.

Study Questions	Key Terms	Suggested Readings
1.a.	Diagnostic Problems in Pediatrics; Development of Hand Skills	Case-Smith—T.O.C.
b.	Diagnostic Problems in Pediatrics; Prewriting and Handwriting Skills	Case-Smith—T.O.C.
c.	Diagnostic Problems in Pediatrics	Case-Smith—T.O.C.
	Session 13/Gross Motor	Scheerer—T.O.C.
d.	Diagnostic Problems in Pediatrics; The Development of Postural Control	Case-Smith—T.O.C.
e.	Diagnostic Problems in Pediatrics; The Development of Postural Control	Case-Smith—T.O.C.
f.	Diagnostic Problems in Pediatrics; Visual Perception	Case-Smith—T.O.C.
g.	Diagnostic Problems in Pediatrics; Feeding and Oral Motor Skills	Case-Smith—T.O.C.
h.	Diagnostic Problems in Pediatrics; Self-care and Adaptations for Independent Living	Case-Smith—T.O.C.
i.	Diagnostic Problems in Pediatrics; Psychosocial and Emotional Domains of Behavior	Case-Smith—T.O.C.

Activity–Teaching Strategies

1. This looks like a relatively short exercise, but it can be quite time-consuming as each student presents. Encourage students to place their handouts in an ongoing reference folder where other intervention ideas can be added. Use the students' presentations for a grade, scoring them on their handouts as well.

Follow-up

Refer to the chart below for the appropriate evaluative source most helpful in assuring that your students integrate the information from this exercise.

Application of Competencies (end of chapter 3 in CCOT)	Performance Skills (end of chapter 3 in CCOT)	Appendix (in CCOT)	Clinical Competency Checklist (appendix in IM)
X	3A		X

Range of Motion

Study Questions–Key Terms/Readings

Use the chart below to find information addressing each study question. Look up the key terms in the sources given in the suggested readings column. Refer to the index, the table of contents (T.O.C.), or other locations as indicated.

Study Questions	Key Terms	Suggested Readings
1.	Range of motion, definition of	Pierson—index
2.	Range of motion, exercises	Pierson—index
3.	Range of motion, exercises	Pierson—index
4.	Evaluation, of hand skill	Case-Smith—index
5.	Upper extremity(ies), passive exercises for	Pierson—index

Activity–Teaching Strategies

1. Review range-of-motion precautions that need to be taken with children such as the presence of pain, fractures, and joint instability. Review pediatric conditions that may need range of motion as a treatment modality. Include diagnoses such as juvenile rheumatoid arthritis, arthrogryposis, and cerebral palsy.

2.a.–c. Demonstrate the proper technique for performing passive, active assistive, and active range of motion. Demonstrate how toys may be used to assist with increasing range of motion. Arrange available toys and positioning equipment around the room, showing the students what is available for them to use. Give feedback to students on their range-of-motion performance as well as their use of the toys and positioning apparatus. Make sure students know each of the movements as well as the normal range for that movement.

3. Begin the "Simon Says . . ." game and then let the students take over. This is a fun way for students to assess their learning and improve their knowledge of the movements involved in range of motion.

Follow-up

Refer to the chart below for the appropriate evaluative source most helpful in assuring that your students integrate the information from this exercise.

Application of Competencies (end of chapter 3 in CCOT)	Performance Skills (end of chapter 3 in CCOT)	Appendix (in CCOT)	Clinical Competency Checklist (appendix in IM)
X			X

Positioning and Handling

Study Questions–Key Terms/Readings

Use the chart below to find information addressing each study question. Look up the key terms in the sources given in the suggested readings column. Refer to the index, the table of contents (T.O.C.), or other locations as indicated.

Study Questions	Key Terms	Suggested Readings
1.	Handling; Positioning, guidelines for	Kramer—index
2.a.–e.	Biomechanical frame of reference, application to practice	Kramer—index
3.	Feeding, positions for oral skills intervention	Case-Smith—index
4.	Handling; Positioning, guidelines for	Kramer—index
5.	Handling; Positioning, guidelines for; Handling, therapeutic, equipment for	Kramer—index
6.	Positioning, for hand skills intervention	Case-Smith—index
7.	Handling; Positioning, guidelines for	Kramer—index
8.	Postulates regarding change, for NeuroDevelopmental Treatment frame of reference	Kramer—index
9.	Postulates regarding change, for NeuroDevelopmental Treatment frame of reference	Kramer—index
10.	Antigravity movement, developmental of	Case-Smith—index
11.	Neurodevelopmental Treatment Frame of Reference	Kramer—T.O.C.
	Motor Learning Theory	Case-Smith—index
12.	Key points of control	Kramer—index
13.	Postural control, intervention and	Case-Smith—index
14.a–e.	Weightbearing and related terms: Weightshifting and related terms	Kramer—index
15.	Proximal key points, handling at	Kramer—index
16.	Antigravity movement, development of	Case-Smith—index
17.	The Development of Postural Control	Case-Smith—T.O.C.

Activity–Teaching Strategies

1. When beginning this activity, start with a very light box. Once everyone has been checked for proper technique, add weights to the box. Alternatively, provide a mannequin for the student's practice. Discuss with the students the importance of preventing injury to their backs. Emphasize the imperativeness of a lifetime of proper lifting habits and the impact these habits will have on their future clinical practice.

---

2. Use several size dolls or mannequins for this demonstration. Students may benefit from several practice sessions. Arrange for children (typical or atypical) to come to the lab as volunteers for the students to practice placing in the positioning devices.

3. Have students practice proper lifting techniques with the large mannequin and with small peers. Check the performances of students as they practice. Provide feedback on accuracy of technique used with each lift performed.

4. Have toys out by the positioning equipment so that once the subject has been positioned the students may simulate an activity using this position. If children are available for demonstration purposes, have the students position them on the equipment. Have students engage the children in a game, noting the changes in positioning over time.

Follow-up

Refer to the chart below for the appropriate evaluative source most helpful in assuring that your students integrate the information from this exercise.

Application of Competencies (end of chapter 3 in CCOT)	Performance Skills (end of chapter 3 in CCOT)	Appendix (in CCOT)	Clinical Competency Checklist (appendix in IM)
X			X

Reflexes

Study Questions–Key Terms/Readings

Use the chart below to find information addressing each study question. Look up the key terms in the sources given in the suggested readings column. Refer to the index, the table of contents (T.O.C.), or other locations as indicated.

Study Questions	Key Terms	Suggested Readings
1.	Primitive reflexes	Case-Smith—index
2.	Primitive reflexes	Case-Smith—index
3.	Primitive reflexes	Case-Smith—index
4.	Reflexes, testing of	Neidstadt—index
5.	Reflexes, testing of	Neidstadt—index

Activity–Teaching Strategies

1. You may wish to demonstrate the testing of the reflexes prior to having the students practice. You may choose to divide up the reflexes and only make the students responsible for learning several and then teaching the one(s) for which they are responsible to the rest of the class.

2. Have several resources available for the students to find this information. One such source is D. B. McCormack's and K. R. Perrin's *Spatial, Temporal, and Physical Analysis of Motor Control: A Comprehensive Guide to Reflexes and Reactions* (San Antonio, TX: Therapy Skill Builders, 1997).

3. If possible, visit a clinic and videotape children who display primitive reflexes and those that display poorly integrated reactions. You may also find a commercially available videotape to use in class.

Follow-up

Refer to the chart below for the appropriate evaluative source most helpful in assuring that your students integrate the information from this exercise.

Application of Competencies (end of chapter 3 in CCOT)	Performance Skills (end of chapter 3 in CCOT)	Appendix (in CCOT)	Clinical Competency Checklist (appendix in IM)
X			

Play

Study Questions–Key Terms/Readings

Use the chart below to find information addressing each study question. Look up the key terms in the sources given in the suggested readings column. Refer to the index, the table of contents (T.O.C.), or other locations as indicated.

Study Questions	Key Terms	Suggested Readings
1.	Reflective	
2.	Play and Occupational Therapy	Parham—T.O.C.
3.	Play, intervention for	Case-Smith—index
4.a.–e.	Play, scope of in pediatric occupational therapy	Case-Smith—index
	Play and Occupational Therapy	Parham—T.O.C.
5.a.–d.	Play, scope of in pediatric occupational therapy; Play, improving skills for	Case-Smith—index
6.a.–e.	Reflective	Labels on toys in toy stores

Activity–Teaching Strategies

1. Distribute identical supplies to each small group of students, for example, shoe box, tennis ball, figures of people and animal, and yarn. Encourage students to come up with the most creative game or activity they can using these materials. Further challenge students by directing them to create a different activity for several different age groups, using the same materials. Discuss the therapeutic implications of the activities.

2.a.–c. As a supplemental activity, have the students observe children at play and record the different levels of ability.

Follow-up

Refer to the chart below for the appropriate evaluative source most helpful in assuring that your students integrate the information from this exercise.

Application of Competencies (end of chapter 3 in CCOT)	Performance Skills (end of chapter 3 in CCOT)	Appendix (in CCOT)	Clinical Competency Checklist (appendix in IM)
X			

Feeding

Study Questions–Key Terms/Readings

Use the chart below to find information addressing each study question. Look up the key terms in the sources given in the suggested readings column. Refer to the index, the table of contents (T.O.C.), or other locations as indicated.

Study Questions	Key Terms	Suggested Readings
1.	Feeding and Oral Motor Skills	Case-Smith—T.O.C.
2.	Conditions Affecting Feeding and Eating	Klein—T.O.C.
	Feeding, sensory defensiveness and	Case-Smith—index
3.	Feeding, nonoral; Feeding, positions for oral skills intervention; Intervention, for self-feeding	Case-Smith—index
4.a.–e.	Oral-Motor Treatment Strategies	Klein—T.O.C.
5.a.–c.	Adaptive equipment, for self feeding	Case-Smith—index
6.	Feeding, handling techniques for	Case-Smith—index
7.	Feeding, handling techniques for	Case-Smith—index
8.	Feeding, handling techniques for	Case-Smith—index
9.	Feeding, handling techniques for	Case-Smith—index
10.a.–b.	Feeding, treatment sequence for	Farber—index
11.	Dysphagia	Reed—index
12.	Intervention, for sensory defensiveness	Case-Smith—index
13.	The Suck/Swallow/Breath Synchrony	Oetter—T.O.C.
14.	The Suck/Swallow/Breath Synchrony	Oetter—T.O.C.
15.	The Suck/Swallow/Breath Synchrony	Oetter—T.O.C.
16.	Treatment Principles and Activities	Oetter—T.O.C.

Activity–Teaching Strategies

1. Discuss conditions such as bite reflex, poor mouth closure, decreased gag reflex, delayed swallow, tongue thrust, and tactile hypersensitivity in and around the mouth. You may demonstrate on a volunteer, doll, or a mannequin. Instruct the students in use and application of rubber gloves and how they should be used in feeding and oral motor techniques. Also discuss universal precautions and demonstrate hand-washing techniques if this has not already been covered in class. Also review the Heimlich maneuver and how it should be used with children in wheelchairs.

2. Have the students feed each with the food that they brought using the improper techniques. Explain to the students that this activity may seem cruel, but that all of these techniques have been observed being done to children and adults being fed by a staff member. It is therefore important to experience the ill effects of these techniques so that each practitioner will be certain to avoid them. Emphasize safety precautions throughout this exercise.

3. Have students feed each other using the food they brought with them. You may wish to have some extra available for those who may have forgotten. As students are practicing these techniques, give them feedback on their techniques.

4. Some students feel more comfortable with one hold versus another when it comes to feeding, yet the child's needs take precedence. Discuss with them the need to experiment with what works best for the client they are feeding.

5. Remind students that the major occupation of children is play and they will want to make certain they incorporate this into their treatment of oral motor deficits, as well as all areas of treatment in pediatrics.

6. Some ideas that students have thought of are passing the pom-poms with the straws by having members hold the pom-pom until it is held by the straw of the person next to them, playing table soccer with the pom-poms and straws by blowing the pom-poms across the table, and sucking through the straws to pick up the pom-poms and place them on a drawn tic tac toe board.

7.a.–c. If a site visit is not possible, obtain a videotape demonstrating various feeding problems and techniques from a colleague.

8. Remind the students to make this fun and encourage creativity.

Follow-up

Refer to the chart below for the appropriate evaluative source most helpful in assuring that your students integrate the information from this exercise.

Application of Competencies (end of chapter 3 in CCOT)	Performance Skills (end of chapter 3 in CCOT)	Appendix (in CCOT)	Clinical Competency Checklist (appendix in IM)
X		B: Therapeutic Use of Self Analysis	X

Hand Skills

Study Questions–Key Terms/Readings

Use the chart below to find information addressing each study question. Look up the key terms in the sources given in the suggested readings column. Refer to the index, the table of contents (T.O.C.), or other locations as indicated.

Study Questions	Key Terms	Suggested Readings
1.a.–d.	Grasp	Case-Smith—index
2.a.–i.	Grasp, classification of	Case-Smith—index
3.a.–f.	Therapeutic Fine-Motor Activities for Preschoolers; Handwriting: Evaluation and Intervention in School Settings	Case-Smith and Pehoski—T.O.C.
4.	Grasp, sequential development of	Case-Smith—index
5.	In-Hand Manipulation Skills	Case-Smith and Pehoski—T.O.C.
	In-hand manipulation, intervention	Case-Smith—index
6.a.–h.	Hand skills, evaluation of	Case-Smith—index
7.a.–d.	In-hand manipulation, treatment activities	Case-Smith—index
8.a.–d.	Hand skills, intervention for	Case-Smith—index
9.	Motor Assessments	Asher—T.O.C.
	Hand skills, evaluation of	Case-Smith—index
	In-Hand Manipulation Skills	Case-Smith and Pehoski—T.O.C.

Activity–Teaching Strategies

1. Alternatively, have students play a game of "Simon Says . . ." having the students do the grasp as Simon instructs and demonstrates. Discuss the development of these grasps along the age line. Draw an age line on the board and have students put the time when each grasp develops. Discuss toys, games, and activities that encourage the use of the different grasps.

2. Videotape children at play and have the tape available for students to watch in addition to visiting a site. Assign students to complete an observation focusing on the children's hand skills on their own initiative and discuss it at a later date.

3. This game may be played individually or with a partner. Following the game, discuss common functional tasks that may not have been mentioned.

Follow-up

Refer to the chart below for the appropriate evaluative source most helpful in assuring that your students integrate the information from this exercise.

Application of Competencies (end of chapter 3 in CCOT)	Performance Skills (end of chapter 3 in CCOT)	Appendix (in CCOT)	Clinical Competency Checklist (appendix in IM)
X			

Handwriting

Study Questions–Key Terms/Readings

Use the chart below to find information addressing each study question. Look up the key terms in the sources given in the suggested readings column. Refer to the index, the table of contents (T.O.C.), or other locations as indicated.

Study Questions	Key Terms	Suggested Readings
1.	View video for content information	Hanft—index
2.	Handwriting, process of	Case-Smith—index
3.	Prewriting and Handwriting Skills	Case-Smith—T.O.C.
4.	Prewriting development	Knight and Decker—T.O.C.
	Handwriting readiness	Case-Smith—index
5.	Therapeutic Fine-Motor Activities for Preschoolers	Case-Smith and Pehoski—T.O.C.
6.	Therapeutic Fine-Motor Activities for Preschoolers	Case-Smith and Pehoski—T.O.C.
7.	Developing Good Habits for Handwriting	Knight and Decker—T.O.C.
8.	Handwriting, instruction methods; Handwriting, intervention for	Case-Smith—index
9.	Handwriting, intervention for	Case-Smith—index
	Handwriting: Evaluation and Intervention in School Settings	Knight and Decker—T.O.C.
10.	Handwriting: Evaluation and Intervention in School Settings	Knight and Decker—T.O.C.
11.	Adaptive equipment, for classroom activities	Case-Smith—index
12.	Handwriting, assessment of	Case-Smith—index
	Handwriting: Evaluation and Intervention in School Settings	Case-Smith and Pehoski—T.O.C.

Activity–Teaching Strategies

1.a.–b. Have students practice administering the Evaluation Tool of Children's Handwriting (Amundson, 1995) following your demonstration. Have students complete an occupational analysis independently or in a small group. Due to the length of this entire exercise, consider giving the occupational analysis as homework assignment or a graded assignment.

2. Place the designated activities around the room in stations. Have students experience each station and then rotate to the next one.

3. Demonstrate the techniques as described by Olsen (1998). Invite a pediatric occupational therapy practitioner or a school-based therapist to demonstrate the

technique for your class. Have students practice using the technique with each other.

4. If you do not have access to a variety of pencil grips, purchase a variety pack that is marketed for evaluative purposes. Allow students to experience a variety of different types of writing paper such as graph paper, raised-line paper, color-coded paper, and so on.

5. Make alphabet posters ahead of time demonstrating how the letters should be formed. Display the posters in the room for the students while they are practicing their letters.

6, 7. Add your own samples of children's handwriting to these.

8. Determine part of the scenario for this child by predetermining the treatment setting, the space and equipment available, the time frame for treatment, and whether the child is seen for intervention in the classroom or pulled out for treatment in a separate space. Give each group a different scenario so when presenting their ideas to the class students will see the difference made by the context setting. Discuss the implementation of a handwriting group and how this child may benefit from such a group. Have the students design a protocol for such a group with this child being one of the founding members.

9. The students should now have many ideas on how to adapt the task of handwriting. Encourage them to add original ideas to those presented in this exercise.

Follow-up

Refer to the chart below for the appropriate evaluative source most helpful in assuring that your students integrate the information from this exercise.

Application of Competencies (end of chapter 3 in CCOT)	Performance Skills (end of chapter 3 in CCOT)	Appendix (in CCOT)	Clinical Competency Checklist (appendix in IM)
X			

Activities of Daily Living

Study Questions–Key Terms/Readings

Use the chart below to find information addressing each study question. Look up the key terms in the sources given in the suggested readings column. Refer to the index, the table of contents (T.O.C.), or other locations as indicated.

Study Questions	Key Terms	Suggested Readings
1.	Self care, importance of	Case-Smith—index
2.	Self care, factors affecting	Case-Smith—index
3.	Self care, intervention for	Case-Smith—index
4.a.–c.	Self care, approaches to improving	Case-Smith—index
5.a.–f.	Self care, intervention for	Case-Smith—index
6.a.–g.	Self care, intervention for	Case-Smith—index
7.	Self care, assessment and	Case-Smith—index
	Assessments (instruments), for children	Neidstadt—index

Activity–Teaching Strategies

1. Discuss situations where forward and backward chaining may be beneficial to use as a teaching tool. Have students draw sequential pictures illustrating the techniques. Have students add color to the pictures and laminate them for future use. Discuss other techniques to assist in improving a child's ADL performance, including the use of adaptive equipment.

2. Discuss the role of the family in this treatment area. Brainstorm play activities that could be used in the treatment of ADLs, for example, dress-up relay races.

Follow-up

Refer to the chart below for the appropriate evaluative source most helpful in assuring that your students integrate the information from this exercise.

Application of Competencies (end of chapter 3 in CCOT)	Performance Skills (end of chapter 3 in CCOT)	Appendix (in CCOT)	Clinical Competency Checklist (appendix in IM)
X			

Adaptations

Study Questions–Key Terms/Readings

Use the chart below to find information addressing each study question. Look up the key terms in the sources given in the suggested readings column. Refer to the index, the table of contents (T.O.C.), or other locations as indicated.

Study Questions	Key Terms	Suggested Readings
1.	Assistive technology (AT), in self-care/IADL	Case-Smith—index
2.	See content area listings	Christensen—entire book Morris—entire book Various adaptive equipment catalogues

Activity–Teaching Strategies

1. Review carefully the chart in study question #2 having the students filling in information they may not have been able to find or think of on their own. Have students use this chart to identify ideas for their case study. Discuss the usefulness of this chart in explaining the parameters of occupational therapy intervention. Have flip charts available for the students to share their information with the class.

2. Provide the class with a case study or problem situation to get them in a creative mode. If possible, have students actually construct their piece of adaptive equipment, either individually or in a small group. Challenge students to actually submit their ideas to a potential manufacturer. Award extra credit points for doing so.

Follow-up

Refer to the chart below for the appropriate evaluative source most helpful in assuring that your students integrate the information from this exercise.

Application of Competencies (end of chapter 3 in CCOT)	Performance Skills (end of chapter 3 in CCOT)	Appendix (in CCOT)	Clinical Competency Checklist (appendix in IM)
X			

Behavior Management

Study Questions–Key Terms/Readings

Use the chart below to find information addressing each study question. Look up the key terms in the sources given in the suggested readings column. Refer to the index, the table of contents (T.O.C.), or other locations as indicated.

Study Questions	Key Terms	Suggested Readings
1.a.	Temperaments, types of	Case-Smith—index
b.	Social skills	Case-Smith—index
c.	Mastering motivation	Case-Smith—index
d.	Self-esteem, as component of social competence	Case-Smith—index
e.	Personal causation	Case-Smith—index
f.	Learned helplessness	Case-Smith—index
2.	Emotional dysfunctions, early signs of	Case-Smith—index
3.a.–h.	Theories, of psychosocial dysfunction	Case-Smith—index
4.	Psychosocial dysfunctions, evaluation of	Case-Smith—index
5.a.–i.	Psychosocial intervention	Case-Smith—index
6.a.–k.	Psychosocial dysfunctions, therapy for disabled children	Case-Smith—index
7.	Psychosocial Dysfunction in Childhood and Adolescence	Neidstadt—T.O.C.
8.	Psychosocial Dysfunction in Childhood and Adolescence	Neidstadt—T.O.C.

Activity–Teaching Strategies

1. Instruct students to use the information in study question #6 for this activity. Once all partners have presented their ideas, have the students select one strategy for each behavior they think likely to be the most effective.

2. Discuss ways to work with the family to improve the child's functioning level. Determine ways to draw on the strengths of families.

3.a.–b. Vote on the best charts and contracts, displaying all of them in the room. Ask the class to critique and share their views on what makes the "winner" a good chart and contract. Have students record some of the ideas from their classmates for future reference.

Follow-up

Refer to the chart below for the appropriate evaluative source most helpful in assuring that your students integrate the information from this exercise.

Application of Competencies (end of chapter 3 in CCOT)	Performance Skills (end of chapter 3 in CCOT)	Appendix (in CCOT)	Clinical Competency Checklist (appendix in IM)
X			

Sensory Integration

Study Questions—Key Terms/Readings

Use the chart below to find information addressing each study question. Look up the key terms in the sources given in the suggested readings column. Refer to the index, the table of contents (T.O.C.), or other locations as indicated.

Study Questions	Key Terms	Suggested Readings
1.a.	Neural plasticity	Fisher—index
b.	Sensory registration disorders	Case-Smith—index
c.	Tactile Processing and Sensory Defensiveness	Fisher—T.O.C.
d.	Hyporesponsivity	Case-Smith—index
e.	Hyperresponsivity	Case-Smith—index
f.	Sensory defensiveness and sensory dormancy	Fisher—index
g.	Sensory discrimination problems	Case-Smith—index
h.	Sensory nourishment	Case-Smith—index
i.	Clinical observation, in sensory integration dysfunction assessment	Case-Smith—index
j.	Sensory integrative dysfunction	Case-Smith—index
k.	Sensory integrative dysfunction, intervention for	Case-Smith—index
l.	Adaptive behavior	Fisher—index
m.	Sensory integrative dysfunction, intervention for, expected outcomes	Case-Smith—index
n.	Sensory integrative dysfunction, assessment of	Case-Smith—index
2.	Group therapy, for sensory integrative intervention	Case-Smith—index
3.a.–d.	Sensory Integration Therapy	Toronto—index
4.	Sensory integrative dysfunction, intervention for	Case-Smith—index
5.	Reflective	
6.	Sensory integrative dysfunction, intervention for	Case-Smith—index
7.	Introduction, Directions, Sensory Input	Scheerer—T.O.C.
8.	Sensory integration (SI) intervention, precautions for	Neidstadt—index
9.	Compensating skills, developing in sensory integrative intervention	Case-Smith—index
10.	Group therapy, for sensory integrative intervention	Case-Smith—index
11.	Consultation, sensory integrative treatment and	Case-Smith—index
12.	Introduction, Current Theory	Scheerer—T.O.C.
13.a.	Session 4/Vestibular System Activities	Scheerer—T.O.C.

(Continues)

Study Questions	Key Terms	Suggested Readings
b.	Session 5/Proprioceptive System	Scheerer—T.O.C.
c.	Session 6/Tactile System	Scheerer—T.O.C.
d.	Intervention; for sensory defensiveness	Case-Smith—Index
e.	Session 3/Oral Motor Needs and Activities	Scheerer—T.O.C.
f.	Session 9/Postural Responses	Scheerer—T.O.C.
g.	Session 10/Ocular Control	Scheerer—T.O.C.
14.	Gravitational insecurity, treatment of, and general guidelines for	Fisher—index
15.	Reflective	

Activity–Teaching Strategies

1. This site visit may need to be planned outside of school hours depending on the availability of the sensory integration clinic. Schedule this visit far in advance so students can make the necessary arrangements to meet after school hours, in the evening, or on the weekend. Emphasize the safety precautions necessary to ensure that no one gets hurt. Discuss the need to respect the differences in individual responses to movement and tactile activities. Have students note any physical effects they experience during their participation in the activities as well as several hours following their participation.

2. Demonstrate all of the techniques. Add your own favorite activities to the list. Be aware of the students in your class who may have some tactile sensitivity or overreactivity issues. Discuss the need to respect each person's tolerance, while also encouraging all students to participate as much as possible so that they will know how it feels to a child with dysfunction.

3. Have students bring the sensory items from home. Encourage creativity and an environment of fun. Have extra tactile items available for use by all groups, such as feathers, lotion, sand, or felt fabric.

4. Have students discuss how their own sensory preferences and tolerances affect their day to day performance. Use the book entitled, "The Out-of-Sync Child: Recognizing and Coping with Sensory Integration Dysfunction" by Carol Stock Kranowitz (1998; The Berkley Publishing Group, New York) as a foundation for this discussion.

Follow-up

Refer to the chart below for the appropriate evaluative source most helpful in assuring that your students integrate the information from this exercise.

Application of Competencies (end of chapter 3 in CCOT)	Performance Skills (end of chapter 3 in CCOT)	Appendix (in CCOT)	Clinical Competency Checklist (appendix in IM)
X			

School-Based Practice

Study Questions–Key Terms/Readings

Use the chart below to find information addressing each study question. Look up the key terms in the sources given in the suggested readings column. Refer to the index, the table of contents (T.O.C.), or other locations as indicated.

Study Questions	Key Terms	Suggested Readings
1.	School-based occupational therapy, legislation related to	Case-Smith—index
2.a.–d.	School-based occupational therapy, process of	Case-Smith—index
3.	School-based occupational therapy, program planning	Case-Smith—index
4.a.–c.	School-based occupational therapy, corrective approach to intervention	Case-Smith—index
5.a.–d.	Compensatory skills, developing in school-based occupational therapy	Case-Smith—index
6.	School-based occupational therapy, integrated vs. pull-out therapy	Case-Smith—index
7.	School-based occupational therapy, integrated vs. pull-out therapy	Case-Smith—index
8.	School-based occupational therapy, collaboration in	Case-Smith—index
	Individual education plans, for transition services	Case-Smith—index
9.	Service delivery, models for, school-based occupational therapy	Case-Smith—index
10.	School-based occupational therapy, process of	Case-Smith—index
11.	Transition services, legislative mandating	Case-Smith—index
12.a.–c.	Transition Services: From School to Adult Life	Case-Smith—T.O.C.
13.	Transition services, legislative mandating	Case-Smith—index
14.	Transition services, legislative mandating	Case-Smith—index
15.a.–c.	Transition services, pediatric occupational therapy in	Case-Smith—index
16.	Sensory Integration Evaluation and Intervention in School-Based Occupation Therapy (1997)	AOTA(latest edition)—T.O.C.

Activity–Teaching Strategies

1.a.–d. Arrange to have all the student complete this observation together or have students initiate individual contact with a school. Organize the observation so that each grade is observed and on completion students learn about the student's tasks across the grade spans.

2. You may provide a list of team members (e.g., principal, teacher, parent, psychiatrist, speech and language pathologist) for the students. Assign each small group a different team member and encourage the students to provide detailed and specific information for that team member. Reconvene small group

members to share with the entire class. Invite one or more team members to share with the students how the team functions in their settings. Invite a school-based therapist to share strategies used when providing school-based intervention.

3.a.–d. Select a job that may be available for a young adult who is developmentally delayed, such as one in the area of food service, office assistance, or cleaning services. Invite an occupational therapy practitioner who works in this type of setting to speak to the students regarding his/her roles in job training and coaching. Have the guest give case and job examples. Allow students time to ask questions regarding this type of setting.

Follow-up

Refer to the chart below for the appropriate evaluative source most helpful in assuring that your students integrate the information from this exercise.

Application of Competencies (end of chapter 3 in CCOT)	Performance Skills (end of chapter 3 in CCOT)	Appendix (in CCOT)	Clinical Competency Checklist (appendix in IM)
X			

Early Intervention

Study Questions–Key Terms/Readings

Use the chart below to find information addressing each study question. Look up the key terms in the sources given in the suggested readings column. Refer to the index, the table of contents (T.O.C.), or other locations as indicated.

Study Questions	Key Terms	Suggested Readings
1.	Early intervention, defined; Early intervention, inclusion model for	Case-Smith—index
2.	Early intervention, required services	Case-Smith—index
3.	Early intervention, IFSPs and	Case-Smith—index
4.	Early intervention, family-centered services and	Case-Smith—index
5.	Evaluation, for early intervention	Case-Smith—index
6.	Evaluation, for early intervention	Case-Smith—index
7.	Teams, for early intervention	Case-Smith—index
8.	Fine motor skills, early intervention for	Case-Smith—index
	Fine motor skills, early intervention for, assessment and	Case-Smith—index
	Play, early intervention and	Case-Smith—index
	Play Assessments	Asher—T.O.C.
	Early intervention, feeding and	Case-Smith—index
	Evaluation, of feeding skills	Case-Smith—index
	Early intervention, sensory integration and	Case-Smith—index
	Evaluation, for early intervention	Case-Smith—index
	Adaptive equipment, early intervention and	Case-Smith—index
	Biomechanical Frame of Reference	Kramer—T.O.C.
	Early intervention, evaluation	Case-Smith—index
	Activities of daily living, pediatric rehabilitation and	Case-Smith—index

Activity–Teaching Strategies

1. Have students try out the toys in a position typically used when playing with the specific toys. Discuss how the toys can be used for intervention. Select a toy and have the class perform an occupational analysis on it.

2. Have students visit a toy store or obtain a toy catalogue. Have students select toy(s) appropriate for each of the following age groups: 0–6 months, 6 months

to 1 year, 1–3 years, 3–5 years, 6–8 years, 9–11 years, and 12–15 years. Discuss possible adaptations for commercially made toys.

Follow-up

Refer to the chart below for the appropriate evaluative source most helpful in assuring that your students integrate the information from this exercise.

Application of Competencies (end of chapter 3 in CCOT)	Performance Skills (end of chapter 3 in CCOT)	Appendix (in CCOT)	Clinical Competency Checklist (appendix in IM)
X			

Hospital Services and Rehabilitation

Study Questions—Key Terms/Readings

Use the chart below to find information addressing each study question. Look up the key terms in the sources given in the suggested readings column. Refer to the index, the table of contents (T.O.C.), or other locations as indicated.

Study Questions	Key Terms	Suggested Readings
1.	Pediatric rehabilitation, teams	Case-Smith—index
2.a.–e.	Hospital, scope of services in	Case-Smith—index
3.	Hospital, pediatric occupational therapy in	Case-Smith—index
4.a.	Burn units, pediatric occupational therapy in	Case-Smith—index
b.	Bone marrow transplant units, pediatric occupational therapy in	Case-Smith—index
c.	Spina bifida	Case-Smith—index
d.	Seizures, epilepsy and	Case-Smith—index
e.	Child abuse, children at risk of	Case-Smith—index
f.	Self-Care Strategies after Spinal Cord Injury	Christiansen—T.O.C.
g.	Traumatic injuries, brain	Case-Smith—index
h.	Brachial plexus injuries, implication for neonatal occupational therapy	Case-Smith—index
i.	Arthrogryposis multiplex congenita	Case-Smith—index
j.	Muscular dystrophies	Case-Smith—index
k.	Juvenile rheumatoid arthritis	Case-Smith—index

Activity—Teaching Strategies

1.a.–e. Have OTA students begin this activity with letter c; have OT students complete all sections. Provide background information for all students, describing how much time the client will have for therapy and what equipment is available in the clinic. Have students plan their treatments, including describing how a OTA and OT would work together on such a case.

2.a.–d. If time allows, have students participate in all three team meetings (initial, progress, and discharge). If time does not allow, select one of the meetings for students to role-play or divide the class into groups and have each group experience one of the different meetings reporting the experience back to the class. Make sure the students include the family in their team meetings.

Follow-up

Refer to the chart below for the appropriate evaluative source most helpful in assuring that your students integrate the information from this exercise.

Application of Competencies (end of chapter 3 in CCOT)	Performance Skills (end of chapter 3 in CCOT)	Appendix (in CCOT)	Clinical Competency Checklist (appendix in IM)
X			

Durable Medical Equipment

Study Questions–Key Terms/Readings

Use the chart below to find information addressing each study question. Look up the key terms in the sources given in the suggested readings column. Refer to the index, the table of contents (T.O.C.), or other locations as indicated.

Study Questions	Key Terms	Suggested Readings
1.	Mobility, developmental theory of	Case-Smith—index
2.	Mobility devices	Case-Smith—index
3.	Durable medical equipment, AAL systems as; Durable medical equipment, mobility and	Case-Smith—index
4.	Mobility devices	Case-Smith—index
5.	Mobility, assessment of	Case-Smith—index
6.	Mobility, assessment of	Case-Smith—index
	Principles of Evaluation	Trefler—T.O.C.
7.	Mobility, assessment of	Case-Smith—index
8.	Rehabilitation technology suppliers, role in mobility assessment	Case-Smith—index
9.	Reflective	
10.	Mobility, assessment of	Case-Smith—index
11.	Wheelchairs	Case-Smith—index
	General Concerns of Seating and Mobility	Trefler—T.O.C.
12.	Mobility devices, factors influencing success of	Case-Smith—index
13.	Mobility devices	Case-Smith—index
	Technology Overview and Classification	Trefler—T.O.C.

Activity–Teaching Strategies

1. Discuss with the durable medical equipment supplier the cost and care of the equipment. Also discuss how frequently insurance companies allow a child to purchase a chair and how a child's growth factor is handled. Have the supplier discuss his or her relationship with occupational therapy in the task of ordering wheelchairs. Have the supplier discuss some of the family's concerns when purchasing a wheelchair for their child.

2. Discuss the pros and cons of each type of walker. Have students simulate a disability while trying out each available type of walker.

3.a.–j. Invite a parent of a child who uses a wheelchair to speak with your class about his or her experiences in both ordering and using a wheelchair with his/her child.

Follow-up

Refer to the chart below for the appropriate evaluative source most helpful in assuring that your students integrate the information from this exercise.

Application of Competencies (end of chapter 3 in CCOT)	Performance Skills (end of chapter 3 in CCOT)	Appendix (in CCOT)	Clinical Competency Checklist (appendix in IM)
X			

Vision Loss and Impairment

Study Questions–Key Terms/Readings

Use the chart below to find information addressing each study question. Look up the key terms in the sources given in the suggested readings column. Refer to the index, the table of contents (T.O.C.), or other locations as indicated.

Study Questions	Key Terms	Suggested Readings
1.	Blindness, defined	Case-Smith—index
2.a.–q.	Visual impairments, diagnosis of	Case-Smith—index
3.a.–e.	Visual impairments, relevance to pediatric occupational therapy	Case-Smith—index
4.	Visual impairments, intervention for	Case-Smith—index
5.	Visual impairments, assessment of	Case-Smith—index
6.a.–n.	Visual impairments, goals/objectives	Case-Smith—index

Activity–Teaching Strategies

1.a.–b. Simulate the experience of a person who is blind trying to recognize unfamiliar objects. Look around your office, classroom, closet, home, and lab for such items, for example, a lock mechanism out of a cabinet or an inside piece to an engine or computer.

2.a.–c. Have students practice using their sense of touch to identify another person as well as experience having to be identified by someone else's sense of touch. Discuss how each student can use a distinctive item when working with a child so that the child can identify them easily. For instance they may wear a certain pin, scarf, or jacket that could easily be identified by the child.

3. Do not allow students to see the projects that they will be working on prior to being blindfolded. Select activities that may be difficult but can be finished fairly quickly such as small leather lacing or making a suncatcher.

4. Allow students to learn by "doing" for this activity. Send them on their way with only basic information about guided walking. They will learn best by experiencing what their partner could have done to be more helpful. If time permits, have them repeat the activity with another partner and compare techniques.

5. If the opportunity exists, take the students to visit a setting that educates children with vision impairments.

6.a.–b. As a supplemental activity, ask the students to spend part of their day using a blindfold to occlude their vision. Have students write in a journal about this experience and share their reactions with the class.

Follow-up

Refer to the chart below for the appropriate evaluative source most helpful in assuring that your students integrate the information from this exercise.

Application of Competencies (end of chapter 3 in CCOT)	Performance Skills (end of chapter 3 in CCOT)	Appendix (in CCOT)	Clinical Competency Checklist (appendix in IM)
X		B: Therapeutic Use of Self-Analysis	

Hearing Loss and Impairment

Study Questions–Key Terms/Readings

Use the chart below to find information addressing each study question. Look up the key terms in the sources given in the suggested readings column. Refer to the index, the table of contents (T.O.C.), or other locations as indicated.

Study Questions	Key Terms	Suggested Readings
1.	Hearing impairments, diagnosis of	Case-Smith—index
2.a.–e.	Hearing impairments, diagnosis of	Case-Smith—index
3.a.–d.	Hearing impairments, intervention for, goals of	Case-Smith—index
4.a.–h.	Hearing aids	Case-Smith—index
5.a.–k.	Total communication	Case-Smith—index
6.	Hearing impairments, assessment of	Case-Smith—index
7.	Hearing impairments, assessment of	Case-Smith—index

Activity–Teaching Strategies

1. Have the audiologist bring hearing aides for children and adults as well. Have the guest discuss communication techniques for students to use when working with a person who is hearing impaired.

2. Obtain sign language cards from a local organization in your community and give each student a copy to keep in his or her wallet. Obtain a poster of the sign language alphabet to display in your classroom. Show a video of basic sign language to your students or have one available in the resource center for them to view at a later date.

3. Pair students who have about the same speed and ability to make the most of this learning experience. Pair those with greater speed and ability with those of lesser speed and ability as a type of tutoring session.

4. Many of the basic signs are in the "Learning the Jargon" exercise found in Chapter One. A local organization may also be able to give you a copy of some of the basic signs used in communication. Discuss the use of sign language in the classrooms.

5. To role-play teaching a child with a severe hearing impairment, have the student who is giving instructions avoid using verbal directions or vocalizations.

Follow-up

Refer to the chart below for the appropriate evaluative source most helpful in assuring that your students integrate the information from this exercise.

Application of Competencies (end of chapter 3 in CCOT)	Performance Skills (end of chapter 3 in CCOT)	Appendix (in CCOT)	Clinical Competency Checklist (appendix in IM)
X			

Working with Families

Study Questions–Key Terms/Readings

Use the chart below to find information addressing each study question. Look up the key terms in the sources given in the suggested readings column. Refer to the index, the table of contents (T.O.C.), or other locations as indicated.

Study Questions	Key Terms	Suggested Readings
1.	Families, defined	Case-Smith—index
2.a.–e.	Families, sources of diversity	Case-Smith—index
3.a.–d.	Families, effect of disabled children on	Case-Smith—index
4.	Family-centered services; Families, communication between therapists and	Case-Smith—index
5.	Culture, effect on families with disabled children	Case-Smith—index

Activity–Teaching Strategies

1.a.–b. Discuss this activity with the families prior to class and have them decide whether they would like to bring their children with them. Having the children present is not necessary but can be an added bonus. Invite families who have children with varying disabilities. If you do not have contacts with families, obtain referrals from your clinical educators, people on your advisory committee, or graduates from your program.

2.a.–c. Role-play the first scenario for the students so they will better understand what you are expecting of them. If students are apprehensive about the experience, have them practice in small groups before doing this assignment in front of the class. Ask the student who is role-playing the occupational therapy practitioner to give feedback on his or her own performance before inviting feedback from others.

Follow-up

Refer to the chart below for the appropriate evaluative source most helpful in assuring that your students integrate the information from this exercise.

Application of Competencies (end of chapter 3 in CCOT)	Performance Skills (end of chapter 3 in CCOT)	Appendix (in CCOT)	Clinical Competency Checklist (appendix in IM)
X	B: Therapeutic Use Of Self-Analysis		

Constructing Assistive Equipment

Study Questions–Key Terms/Readings

Use the chart below to find information addressing each study question. Look up the key terms in the sources given in the suggested readings column. Refer to the index, the table of contents (T.O.C.), or other locations as indicated.

Study Questions	Key Terms	Suggested Readings
1.	Assistive technology (AT), in self-care/IADL	Case-Smith—index
2.	Battery-operated device, selection of	Ryan(a)—index
3.	Battery-operated device, patient treatment applications	Ryan(a)—index
4.	Battery-operated device, safety precautions	Ryan(a)—index
5.a.–d.	Reflective	

Activity–Teaching Strategies

1. Discuss safety precautions that need to be followed when using power equipment. Have students remove any dangling jewelry and make sure their hair is secured back away from their faces so that it will not interfere with the operation of the equipment. Emphasize the need to go slow when using the equipment. Have students work in pairs so they can assist each other in their adherence to safety precautions.

2.a.–b. Allow approximately one and one-half hours to assemble the notebook switches. Have materials readily available for more efficient use of time. Show the students several types of commercially available pressure switches. Provide catalogues for the students to see the types of switches available for children to give them additional ideas. Have students compare the price of a commercially made switch to that of their home-made one.

3.a.–b. If students are doing their pediatric fieldwork at this time, have them ask their facility what piece of equipment they might need. Have the students donate the completed piece of equipment to their facility. If the students are not on clinical rotations at this time, ask several facilities in the community to determine if there is a need for any specific equipment. Have students donate their pieces of adaptive equipment to the various facilities as a way of providing a community service.

Follow-up

Refer to the chart below for the appropriate evaluative source most helpful in assuring that your students integrate the information from this exercise.

Application of Competencies (end of chapter 3 in CCOT)	Performance Skills (end of chapter 3 in CCOT)	Appendix (in CCOT)	Clinical Competency Checklist (appendix in IM)
X	3B, 3C	B: Analysis of Self	X

Pediatric Intervention Planning

Study Questions—Key Terms/Readings

Use the chart below to find information addressing each study question. Look up the key terms in the sources given in the suggested readings column. Refer to the index, the table of contents (T.O.C.), or other locations as indicated.

Study Questions	Key Terms	Suggested Readings
1.	Standards of Practice for Occupational Therapy	AOTA(latest edition)—T.O.C.
2.	Goodness of fit	Case-Smith—index
3.	Intervention plans	Case-Smith—index
4.	Client-centered activities	Case-Smith—index
5.	Teams, problem solving by	Case-Smith—index
6.	Service delivery, models for	Case-Smith—index
7.	Intervention plans, process of	Case-Smith—index
8.	Standards of Practice for Occupational Therapy	AOTA(latest edition)—T.O.C.

Activity—Teaching Strategies

1.a.–h. Have the students do this activity once for practice. Simulate the managed care arena by having students complete this assignment in class, submitting it to be graded as part of the course. Have students complete this assignment toward the end of a course to give them an opportunity to incorporate all the information they have learned to date.

Follow-up

Refer to the chart below for the appropriate evaluative source most helpful in assuring that your students integrate the information from this exercise.

Application of Competencies (end of chapter 3 in CCOT)	Performance Skills (end of chapter 3 in CCOT)	Appendix (in CCOT)	Clinical Competency Checklist (appendix in IM)
X	3E		X

Wellness/Prevention for the Adolescent

Study Questions–Key Terms/Readings

Use the chart below to find information addressing each study question. Look up the key terms in the sources given in the suggested readings column. Refer to the index, the table of contents (T.O.C.), or other locations as indicated.

Study Questions	Key Terms	Suggested Readings
1.a.–c.	Reflective	
2.	Reflective	
3.	Adolescence, development in	Case-Smith—index
4.	Adolescence, families with disabled children and	Case-Smith—index
5.	Adolescence, development in	Case-Smith—index
6.	Adolescence, psychosocial development in	Case-Smith—index

Activity–Teaching Strategies

1.a.–h. Have students prepare to actually give their presentation to a group of adolescents. Make prior arrangements to fill an existing need at a local high school(s) or youth group(s) in the community. Encourage students to initiate their own contact in the community and make arrangements accordingly. Alternatively, have students complete this presentation for each other and simulate an adolescent audience.

Follow-up

Refer to the chart below for the appropriate evaluative source most helpful in assuring that your students integrate the information from this exercise.

Application of Competencies (end of chapter 3 in CCOT)	Performance Skills (end of chapter 3 in CCOT)	Appendix (in CCOT)	Clinical Competency Checklist (appendix in IM)
X		B: Therapeutic Use of Self-Analysis B: Analysis of Self	X

Section Three

Performance Skill 3A

Standardized Testing

Make arrangements with the day care center in your facility or a local community facility to provide children for this standardized testing. Of course, you will need to work out permissions for this activity and have the parents approve any interactions that will occur between their child and your students. Many parents are willing to participate if they understand that their child is simply needed to give students a chance to practice newly acquired skills.

Performance Skill 3B

Toy Adaptation

Have the students do this toy adaptation for a child they are working with at their fieldwork site or one you have assigned. If possible, have them make it for a child they will see on a continuing basis so that the necessary adjustments, corrections, or reworking of the adaptation can be easily made. If the students are not on fieldwork, solicit a volunteer from the community. Most parents and the child or children will be excited to have toys adapted as long as they get to keep them. Encourage students to be creative in their search for toys and adaptations while trying to keep the costs as economical as possible. Discuss local resources that have toys at a reduced price such as garage and yard sales. Have students clean out their own or their friend's closets obtaining toys with which their children no longer play.

Performance Skill 3C

Adaptive Equipment Construction

Have the students make the adaptive equipment for the child to increase independence or to allow the caregiver more ease in caring for the child. For instance, for a child who lacks range of motion in the arms and is unable to assist in caring for him- or herself, an adaptive shirt that opens in the back allowing the caregiver to put the shirt on, would be appropriate. Select clients to whom the adaptive equipment may be given as outlined in the previous Performance Skill 3B.

Performance Skill 3D

Adding to Your Files

Add more targeted areas or suggest that students design the activities specific to a particular setting. Designate the setting and the available equipment. Have students come up with an activity for each of the components working only with the materials and space you have specified. If in your community most pediatric treatment is done in the classroom and not in a separate clinic, have your students focus on this aspect with their files. Alternatively, give the students a budget with which to work. Have them make a treatment box with materials in it to work on all of the treatment components listed. If any of your students plan to work in pediatrics he or she will certainly not mind spending the money and will have a traveling box of treatment activities available for use. Keep in mind that all students are on a limited budget, though, so encourage them to be thrifty and work together in groups, or provide this treatment box assignment as an alternative to the written activity file.

Performance Skill 3E	**Intervention Planning**

Have students complete this performance skill at home or as an in-class assignment. Select any of the cases in the back of this section or generate one of your own. A supervisor may be willing to share referral information on a case (while still maintaining confidentiality) for students to use. Provide OTA student with the initial evaluation and treatment plan. Have them begin with planning treatment activities and revise goals as the client makes improvements.

References

American Occupational Therapy Associations. latest edition. *Reference Manual of the Official Documents of the American Occupational Therapy Association.* Bethesda, MD: Author.

American Occupational Therapy Associations. 1998. *Reference Manual of the Official Documents of the American Occupational Therapy Association.* Bethesda, MD: Author.

Amundson, S. J. 1995. *Evaluation Tool of Children's Handwriting.* Homer, AK: O. T. Kids.

Asher, I. E. 1996. *Occupational Therapy Assessment Tools: An Annotated Index.* 2d ed. Bethesda, MD: American Occupational Therapy Association.

Baker, M., and J. Kilburn. 1992. *Tri-Wall Pattern Portfolio.* Tucson, AZ: Therapy Skill Builders.

Beery, K. E. 1989. *Beery Development Test of Visual Motor Integration.* 3d rev. Cleveland, OH: Modern Curriculum Press.

Bruininks, R. 1978. *Bruininks-Osentesky Test of Motor Proficiency.* Circle Pines, MN: American Guidance Service.

Burkhart, L. J. 1985. *More Homemade Battery Devices for Severely Handicapped with Suggested Activities.* Handout from Assistive Technologist.

Case-Smith, J., A. S. Allen, and P. N. Pratt. 1996. *Occupational Therapy for Children.* 3d ed. St. Louis; Mosby.

Case-Smith, J., and C. Pehoski. 1992. *Development of Hand Skills in the Child.* Bethesda, MD: American Occupational Therapy Association.

Christiansen, C., ed. 2000. *Ways of Living: Self-Care Strategies for Special Needs.* 2d ed. Bethesda, MD: American Occupational Therapy Association.

Costello, E. 1994. *Random House American Sign Language Dictionary.* New York: Random House.

Dunn, W., ed. 1991. *Pediatric Occupational Therapy: Facilitating Effective Service Provision.* Thorofare, NJ: Slack.

Farber, S. D. 1982. *Neurorehabilitation: A Multisensory Approach.* Philadelphia: W. B. Saunders.

Fisher, A. G., E. A. Murray, and A. C. Bundy. 1991. *Sensory Integration Theory and Practice.* Philadelphia: F. A. Davis.

Frankenburg, W. K. 1990. *Denver II: Training Video.* Denver: CO: Denver Developmental Materials.

Frankenburg, W. K., J. Dodds, P. Archer, B. Bresnick, P. Maschka, N. Edelman, and H. Shapiro. 1992. *Denver II Training Manual.* Denver, CO: Denver Developmental Materials.

Hanft, B., and D. Marsh, 1992. *Getting a Grip on Handwriting.* Bethesda, MD: American Occupational Therapy Association.

Henry, D. (n.d.). *Tools for Teachers: A Video on Practical Occupational Therapy Strategies.* Phoenix, AZ: Henry Occupational Therapy Services.

Hinojosa, J., and P. Kramer. 1998. *Evaluation: Obtaining and Interpreting Data.* Sterling, VA: World Composition Services.

Klein, M. D., and T. A. Delaney. 1994. *Feeding and Nutrition for the Child with Special Needs.* Tucson, AZ: Therapy Skill Builders.

Knight, J. M., and M. J. Decker. 1994. *Hands at Work and Play: Developing Fine Motor Skills at School and Home.* Tucson, AZ: Therapy Skill Builders.

Korb-Khalsa, K. L., S. D. Azok, and E. A. Leutenberg. 1995a. *Life Management Skills III.* Beechwood, OH: Wellness Reproductions.

Korb-Khalsa, K. L., S. D. Azok, and E. A. Leutenberg. 1995b. *S.E.A.L.S. + Plus.* Beechwood, OH: Wellness Reproductions.

Kramer, P., and J. Hinojosa. 1998. *Frames of Reference for Pediatric Occupational Therapy.* 2d ed. Baltimore: Lippincott Williams & Wilkins.

Morris, G. S., and D. J. Stiehl. 1989. *Changing Kid's Games.* Champaign, IL: Human Kinetics.

Neidstadt, M. E., and E. B. Crepeau. 1998. *Willard and Spackman's Occupational Therapy.* 9th ed. Philadelphia: J. B. Lippincott.

Oetter, P., E. W. Richter, and S. M. Frick. 1995. *M.O.R.E. Integrating the Mouth with Sensory and Postural Functions.* 2d ed. Hugo, MN: PDP Press.

Olsen, J. S. 1998. *Handwriting Without Tears.* 7th ed. Potomac, MD: Handwriting Without Tears.

Parham, D. L., and L. S. Fazio. 1997. *Play in Occupational Therapy.* St. Louis: Mosby.

Pierson, F. M. 1999. *Principles and Techniques of Patient Care.* 2d ed. Philadelphia: W. B. Saunders.

Reed, K. L. 1991. *Quick Reference to Occupational Therapy.* Gaithersburg, MD: Aspen Publishers.

Ryan, S. E. 1995a. *The Certified Occupational Therapy Assistant: Principles, Concepts, and Techniques.* 2d ed. Thorofare, NJ: Slack.

Scheerer, C. R. 1997. *Sensimotor Groups: Activities for School and Home.* San Antonio, TX: Therapy Skill Builders.

Sher, B. 1992. *Extraordinary Play with Ordinary Things.* Tucson, AZ: Therapy Skill Builders.

Toronto Sensory Integration Group. 1987. *Sensory Integration Therapy.* Tucson, AZ: Therapy Skill Builders.

Trefler, E., D. A. Hobson, S. J. Taylor, L. C. Monahan, and C. G. Shaw. 1993. *Seating and Positioning for Persons with Physical Disabilities.* Tucson, AZ: Therapy Skill Builders.

Observation Skills

Study Questions–Key Terms/Readings

Use the chart below to find information addressing each study question. Look up the key terms in the sources given in the suggested readings column. Refer to the index, the table of contents (T.O.C.), or other locations as indicated.

Study Questions	Key Terms	Suggested Readings
1.	Verbal Communication; Nonverbal Communication	Purtillo–T.O.C.
2.	Listening, blocking to	Denton–index
3.	Observation	Mosey–index
4.a.–c.	Observation, naturalistic	Denton–index
5.	Listening, improvement of	Denton–index
6.	Observation, informal	Early–index
7.	Evaluation, sequence	Mosey–index
8.	Culture, Bias, and Discrimination	Purtillo–T.O.C.

Activity–Teaching Strategies

1. Bring enough oranges (or use other food items that are visually similar) so that each student can select one. Give students a 5-minute time limit to study their oranges. Encourage them to note the specific details of their oranges either mentally or in writing. Then collect the oranges and at a later time (at the end of the class session, for example) have students identify their oranges from the collection.

2. Make this into a game with the "winners" being the ones who can identify all the changes. Encourage students to make obvious changes at first, such as removing eyeglasses. Play the game again with students making more subtle changes, such as slightly rolling up a shirtsleeve.

3.a.–g. This game helps the students get in touch with some of the issues people with mental illness have to face on a daily basis. Getting in touch with client's issues occurs while observing behaviors of the other game players. If you have too many students to play the game, have several observers and then rotate them into playing while others take turns sitting out. In the discussion that follows the game, compare the student's personal experience in playing the game with a real-life clinic setting.

4.a. Writing clear observations makes the task of goal writing much easier.

4.b. A problem statement and goal for the example given in 4a (a behavior not observable or measurable) may read," Client has low self esteem," and "Increase client's self esteem," respectively. Point out to students that a goal written in this manner is not measurable.

4.c. A problem statement and goal for the 2nd observation in 4a would be, "Client has poor grooming skills as demonstrated by wearing soiled clothing to group," and "Client will come to group with clean clothing given one verbal reminder." Point out the case with which this goal could be measured.

4.d. Point out the strong correlation between the ease with which a measurable goal can be made from a measurable observation.

5. Have a student role-play the therapist's role trying to engage you (the client) in an activity such as playing cards. As the therapist relates to you, exhibit the following symptoms for the students to observe: poor eye contact, poor self-esteem, tremors, poor fine-motor coordination, poor bilateral integration, poor sequencing, poor memory, and the like. As an alternative to individual work, have students work in pairs to complete the form.

6. Due to the length of the observation and time constraints, have students discuss their observations in small groups rather than as a large group.

7. The necessity of having good observation skills will be obvious as students attempt to find their original orange. End the class by encouraging students to eat the nutritious treat.

Follow-up

Refer to the chart below for the appropriate evaluative source most helpful in assuring that your students integrate the information from this exercise.

Application of Competencies (end of chapter 4 in CCOT)	Performance Skills (end of chapter 4 in CCOT)	Appendix (in CCOT)	Clinical Competency Checklist (appendix in IM)
X			

Evaluation of Psychosocial Functioning

Study Questions–Key Terms/Readings

Use the chart below to find information addressing each study question. Look up the key terms in the sources given in the suggested readings column. Refer to the index, the table of contents (T.O.C.), or other locations as indicated.

Study Questions	Key Terms	Suggested Readings
1.	Evaluation and assessment of person with psychosocial dysfunction, overview, purpose of testing	Stein—index
2.	Evaluation and assessment of person with psychosocial dysfunction, methods of occupational therapy evaluation	Stein—index
3.	Evaluation and assessment of person with psychosocial dysfunction, test summaries of commonly used tests in psychosocial practice	Stein—index
	Comprehensive Occupational Therapy Evaluation	Asher—index
4.a.–i.	Evaluation and assessment of person with psychosocial dysfunction, methods of occupational therapy evaluation	Stein—index
5.	Comprehensive case study analysis, outline of	Stein—index
6.	Evaluation and assessment of person with psychosocial dysfunction, test summaries of commonly used tests in psychosocial practice	Stein—index
7.	Evaluation, environment	Mosey—index
8.	An Introduction to the Integrative Approach to Mental Health Assessment	Hemphill—T.O.C.
9.	Interview	Mosey—index
10.	Evaluation of Performance Contexts	Neidstadt—T.O.C.
11.a.–e.	Reflective	
12.	Interview, content	Mosey—index
13.	Evaluation and assessment of person with psychosocial dysfunction, module for learning test administration	Stein—index
14.	Functional assessment	Hemphill—index

Activity–Teaching Strategies

1.a. After demonstrating proper test administration techniques, have the tests set up in stations so students can rotate from station to station. Observe, answer questions, and give feedback as necessary.

1.b. Assist students in planning strategies to improve. Schedule open lab times with the tests available for students to practice. Having students practice with and without your presence are both helpful strategies.

1.c. Discuss the percentage of interrater reliability agreement and degree of service competency as ways to determine if a OTA may perform a test.

1.d. List all tests given and whether it is appropriate for a OTA to administer them. Discuss how the students came to their conclusions using the criteria mentioned in 1.c. to assist you. Point out the OTA's role in administering standardized tests and the OT's role in supervising the OTA when contributing to other nonstandardized aspects of the evaluation process.

2. See the sources listed under the suggested reading materials for reference to nonstandardized tests.

Follow-up

Refer to the chart below for the appropriate evaluative source most helpful in assuring that your students integrate the information from this exercise.

Application of Competencies (end of chapter 4 in CCOT)	Performance Skills (end of chapter 4 in CCOT)	Appendix (in CCOT)	Clinical Competency Checklist (appendix in IM)
X		B: Therapeutic Use of Self-Analysis	

Listening and Responding

Study Questions–Key Terms/Readings

Use the chart below to find information addressing each study question. Look up the key terms in the sources given in the suggested readings column. Refer to the index, the table of contents (T.O.C.), or other locations as indicated.

Study Questions	Key Terms	Suggested Readings
1.	Therapeutic Use of Self	Early–T.O.C.
2.	Concreteness	Cole–index
3.	Primary accurate empathy; Advanced accurate empathy	Cole–index
4.	Immediacy	Cole–index
5.	Confrontation	Cole–index
6.	Reflective	
7.a.–j.	Responding to Symptoms and Behaviors	Early–T.O.C.
8.	Interviewing as an Assessment Tool in Occupational Therapy	Hemphill–T.O.C.

Activity–Teaching Strategies

1. Help students understand that one word cannot always describe how a person feels. The more specifically the feeling is described, the more the communicative intent is understood.

2. Help students see the importance of validating another's feelings rather than presuming the feelings from the individual's behavior. Continue the charades as long as time permits. Keep score and award small prizes to the winning team.

3.a.–i. Remind students there is not just one right or wrong answer but many ways to respond that may be appropriate. Given just one statement, it is impossible to know exactly what has been happening. Have students come up with one *possible* reason and how they would respond. The first few may be completed together.

4.a.–b. Have students write about an experience with some emotional attachment to it. Have them practice responding to each other in an empathetic manner, checking for the feelings of the person with whom they are interacting. Discuss how this technique may be helpful not just with clients but in everyday relationships as well.

Follow-up

Refer to the chart below for the appropriate evaluative source most helpful in assuring that your students integrate the information from this exercise.

Application of Competencies (end of chapter 4 in CCOT)	Performance Skills (end of chapter 4 in CCOT)	Appendix (in CCOT)	Clinical Competency Checklist (appendix in IM)
X		B: Therapeutic Use of Self-Analysis	

Interview Process

Study Questions–Key Terms/Readings

Use the chart below to find information addressing each study question. Look up the key terms in the sources given in the suggested readings column. Refer to the index, the table of contents (T.O.C.), or other locations as indicated.

Study Questions	Key Terms	Suggested Readings
1.	Interviewing as an Assessment Tool in Occupational Therapy	Hemphill—T.O.C.
2.	Initial interview, purpose of	Stein—index
3.	Interviewing methods	Early—index
4.	Interviewing methods	Early—index
5.	Initial interview, therapeutic techniques during	Stein—index
6.	Interviewing methods	Early—index
7.	Occupational History interview; Occupational History Interview Illustrated	Early—index
8.	Interviews structure and control of	Hemphill—index
9.	Interviewing as an Assessment Tool in Occupational Therapy	Hemphill—T.O.C.
10.a.–d.	The Occupational Therapy Process: The Basis for Achieving Positive Mental Health Goals	Stein—T.O.C.
11.a.–b.	Questions, format of	Denton—index
12.a.–b.	Questions, format of	Denton—index
13.	Initial interview, therapeutic techniques during	Stein—index
14.	Frame of reference, in data base establishment	Denton—index

Activity–Teaching Strategies

1. Remind students that open-ended questions generally begin with the words "what" or "how" and less frequently with the word "why."

2. Emphasize the importance of establishing rapport. Role-play the difference in a client's cooperativeness or willingness to communicate when time is taken to carefully establish rapport and when it is not.

3. Assist with time management making sure the groups move along and that everyone gets a chance to conduct an interview. Encourage students to give their peers constructive criticism. Remind them that they are helping each other become more skilled at interviewing. The more specific the feedback, the more helpful it is.

4. Videotape in a room apart from where the critiquing occurs. Encourage students to seek as much input as possible from other students. Other students can learn from watching videotapes of interviews in which they did not participate and can assist in the critiquing. Recruit an "outside" or neutral person to perform the client role for the students. Ask your institution for assistance from the drama department or solicit the talent of someone who enjoys acting.

Follow-up

Refer to the chart below for the appropriate evaluative source most helpful in assuring that your students integrate the information from this exercise.

Application of Competencies (end of chapter 4 in CCOT)	Performance Skills (end of chapter 4 in CCOT)	Appendix (in CCOT)	Clinical Competency Checklist (appendix in IM)
X	4B	B: Therapeutic Use of Self-Analysis	X

Assertiveness

Study Questions–Key Terms/Readings

Use the chart below to find information addressing each study question. Look up the key terms in the sources given in the suggested readings column. Refer to the index, the table of contents (T.O.C.), or other locations as indicated.

Study Questions	Key Terms	Suggested Readings
1.a.–c.	Assertiveness; Aggressive behavior; Nonassertive behavior	Davis—index
2.	Personal rights	Davis—index
3.	Attribution theory	Davis—index
4.	Assertive behavior, development	Davis—index
5.a.–d.	DESC response, assertive communication	Davis—index
6.	I statements	Davis—index
7.	Anger, assertively handling	Davis—index
8.	Assertiveness, benefits	Davis—index
9.	Assertiveness training, anxiety disorders and	Cara—index
10.a.–e.	Reflective	
11.	Reflective	

Activity–Teaching Strategies

1.a. Encourage students to describe occupational therapy related scenarios they may have encountered when volunteering, on their field work assignment, or in the classroom.

1.b. Students often view assertive behavior as being aggressive until both behaviors are demonstrated. For example someone saying, "Don't touch me," in a firm manner might be considered assertive whereas saying, "Don't touch me, you're disgusting!" might be considered aggressive. Demonstrate the DESC format to clarify this common misunderstanding. Coach students until they fully understand the differences in the three communication styles. Demonstrate the behaviors as needed.

2. Encourage students to write measurable goals to improve their assertiveness skills as part of their professional behavior development. Let students know that if they are not assertive, it is their clients who will most often lose. They will need to be able to stand up for their clients in team meetings and to those persons in positions of authority to ensure that their clients receive best-practice services. Such an explanation will often help the reluctant student realize

why it is so important to learn assertive behavior. A personal lesson can be learned here as well and the benefits to oneself, and one's profession not only one's clients, can be discussed.

3. Have students write their scenarios about situations in which they project clients may have difficulties.

Follow-up

Refer to the chart below for the appropriate evaluative source most helpful in assuring that your students integrate the information from this exercise.

Application of Competencies (end of chapter 4 in CCOT)	Performance Skills (end of chapter 4 in CCOT)	Appendix (in CCOT)	Clinical Competency Checklist (appendix in IM)
X		B: Therapeutic Use of Self-Analysis	

Social Skills

Study Questions–Key Terms/Readings

Use the chart below to find information addressing each study question. Look up the key terms in the sources given in the suggested readings column. Refer to the index, the table of contents (T.O.C.), or other locations as indicated.

Study Questions	Key Terms	Suggested Readings
1.	Role acquisition	Mosey–index
2.	Social skills training	Cotrell–index
3.a.–j.	Role acquisition, theoretical base	Mosey–index
4.	Social skills training, definition of	Stein–index
5.a.	Attention-focusing skills training model; Social skills training, problem solving model	Cotrell–index
b.	Social skills training	Cotrell–index
6.	Social skills training, generalization; Social skills training, maintenance	Cotrell–index
7.	Social, interaction domains and skills	Cara–index
8.	Culture, spectrum of values	Cara–index
9.	Social skills training, assessments	Stein–index
10.	Reflective	

Activity–Teaching Strategies

1. Discuss with the students the different roles for which they are responsible. Have students reflect how their roles have and will continue to change over the course of their lifetime. Have students compare and contrast their roles with their classmates.

2.a.–c. Social skills/issues that may surface may include, but are certainly not limited to, the following "truisms": do not talk back to authority; speak only when spoken to; it is better to be seen and not heard; if you don't have anything nice to say, don't say anything at all. Reassure students that there is no such thing as a perfect family and that all families have room for improvement. On the chalkboard, list the different cultures represented by the students' families. Have students list characteristics that were or are important to their families under the subheading of their specific culture. Discuss with the class the influences of culture as it relates to social skills. Assist students in identifying those characteristics they want to keep and those with which they want to do away.

3.a.–b. To observe social conduct and interpersonal skills, any controversial topic (spanking, abortion, euthanasia, gun control, etc.) may be used to facilitate a discussion. Have the group(s) select such a topic.

4.a.–c. Check the knot to make sure it is tied correctly. It is most important to be sure that each student has the hand of two different students and not the two hands of the same person. As the class begins problem solving, observe the social skills used by each member. Use this information to facilitate the discussion after the knot is untied. Videotape the group and have students observe their own performance just prior to the discussion. Divide a large group of students into two smaller ones (no smaller than six students to a group), encouraging a little competition as each group races to be the first group to untie the knot. Assure students that most knots can be untied.

5. Select a variety of different social activities with some requiring mostly verbal skills and others requiring more physical contact. Many ideas can be found in Rider and Rider (1999). Select activities that may be useful in chronic, acute, geriatric, and adolescence psychiatric settings.

6. Have flip charts on which students can write their ideas set up in the room. Have the entire class do all of the case studies or assign one to each group and have the different groups share their ideas with the entire class.

Follow-up

Refer to the chart below for the appropriate evaluative source most helpful in assuring that your students integrate the information from this exercise.

Application of Competencies (end of chapter 4 in CCOT)	Performance Skills (end of chapter 4 in CCOT)	Appendix (in CCOT)	Clinical Competency Checklist (appendix in IM)
X			

Cognitive Disability

Study Questions–Key Terms/Readings

Use the chart below to find information addressing each study question. Look up the key terms in the sources given in the suggested readings column. Refer to the index, the table of contents (T.O.C.), or other locations as indicated.

Study Questions	Key Terms	Suggested Readings
1.	Cognitive disabilities, task performance skills	Early—index
2.	Allen, Claudia, theory of cognitive disabilities	Early—index
3.	Allen, Claudia, theory of cognitive disabilities	Early—index
4.	Modes of Performance within the Cognitive Levels	Allen—T.O.C.
5.	Cognitive disability, theory applicability of	Cara—index
6.a.–c.	Responding to Symptoms and Behaviors	Early—T.O.C.
7.a.–e.	Allen Cognitive Level Test	Asher—index
8.	Cognitive disability, theory	Cara—index
9.	Reflective	

Activity–Teaching Strategies

1. Show the video entitled *Administering the ACLS (Allen Cognitive Level Screen)* (available from Allen Conferences, Inc., Ormand Beach, FL, n.d.) to assist students in their preparation of administering the screening tool. Use the larger ACL screening test (Allen, 1992) for demonstration purposes. Ask for a volunteer to complete the assessment and assure the class that many people typically function below a 6.0 level. Ultimate performance on a routine basis is not expected.

2. Invite a group of students who are more advanced in their OT education to come and administer the screening test to the students in your class. Explain the benefits of learning how to administer the test in this way plus the added benefit of a student obtaining insight about his or her own cognitive level. Knowing and understanding this information will assist students in selecting meaningful learning strategies for themselves in the future. Have the students continue to practice with each other until they are able to give the test competently.

3. Along with the mode, include a behavioral description on the index card to familiarize students with behavior typical of that mode. For the first several ex-

examples on the card describing how the student might execute that mode during the ribbon card assembly.

4.a.–b. Have students write goals for their case studies. Ask the students to predict the client's discharge potential and justify their predictions.

Follow-up

Refer to the chart below for the appropriate evaluative source most helpful in assuring that your students integrate the information from this exercise.

Application of Competencies (end of chapter 4 in CCOT)	Performance Skills (end of chapter 4 in CCOT)	Appendix (in CCOT)	Clinical Competency Checklist (appendix in IM)
X	4E		X

Daily Living Skills

Study Questions–Key Terms/Readings

Use the chart below to find information addressing each study question. Look up the key terms in the sources given in the suggested readings column. Refer to the index, the table of contents (T.O.C.), or other locations as indicated.

Study Questions	Key Terms	Suggested Readings
1.	Activities of daily living evaluation, content of	Neidstadt–index
2.	Activities of daily living evaluation, content of	Neidstadt–index
3.	Activities of Daily Living	Early–T.O.C.
4.	Case management, daily living skills development	Cara–index
5.	Activities of daily living evaluation	Neidstadt–index
6.	Activities of daily living evaluation	Neidstadt–index

Activity–Teaching Strategies

1. Have the suggested settings listed on the board or on flip charts located around the room. Have each group start on a setting and rotate to the next one, adding to the list as they go. Keep the needs on display for use in activity #2.

2. Do this in small groups instead of with partners to enable all students to have a turn leading their group. Assign the settings to the students or allow them to choose. Lead the postgroup discussion in a small group setting or with the entire class.

Follow-up

Refer to the chart below for the appropriate evaluative source most helpful in assuring that your students integrate the information from this exercise.

Application of Competencies (end of chapter 4 in CCOT)	Performance Skills (end of chapter 4 in CCOT)	Appendix (in CCOT)	Clinical Competency Checklist (appendix in IM)
X			

Movement

Study Questions–Key Terms/Readings

Use the chart below to find information addressing each study question. Look up the key terms in the sources given in the suggested readings column. Refer to the index, the table of contents (T.O.C.), or other locations as indicated.

Study Questions	Key Terms	Suggested Readings
1.	Movement, traditional treatment; assumptions of	Christiansen–index
	Movement and Touch Related to Neurophysiological Principles	Ross–T.O.C.
2.	Movement; assessment	Christiansen–index
3.	Theories about Exercise and Neurotransmitters	Christiansen–T.O.C.
4.a.–e.	Promoting Health and Physical Fitness	Christiansen–T.O.C.
5.	Promoting Health and Physical Fitness	Christiansen–T.O.C.
6.	Promoting Health and Physical Fitness	Christiansen–T.O.C.
7.	Movement-centered frame of reference, therapist role in	Bruce–index
8.	Movement-centered frame of reference, treatment	Bruce–index
9.	Sensory motor approaches, group treatment	Cole–index
	Promoting Health and Physical Fitness	Christiansen–T.O.C.
	Movement-centered frame of reference, dysfunction in	Bruce–index
10.	King, L. J., sensory motor approaches	Cole–index
11.	Sensory integration (SI) intervention, precautions for	Neidstadt–index
12.a.–c.	Reflective	

Activity–Teaching Strategies

1. Lead at least a half-hour movement group with the students as your members. Prior to starting the group, discuss the age group and the setting for which this group would be appropriate: adolescence, adult, or geriatric, and acute or chronic. As an alternative to leading a typical movement group, select various media and present several movement activities in order to expose the students to a wider variety of movement options. The following examples may be incorporated into your movement group:

   - Warm up by stretching, then doing simple exercises. Have each student take a turn selecting a stretch or exercise as you go around the circle.

   - Play a tape of "oldies" music. Have students sit in chairs in a circle, taking turns being a leader and selecting a movement that coordinates with the music. Direct students to imitate the movement of the leader for about 15 to 30 seconds then continue as the next person selects a movement to lead that coordinates with the next song.

- Play a ball juggling game by tossing the ball to someone after you call his or her name. That person, in turn, then calls a name and tosses the ball to that person. Once everyone has had his or her name called and received the ball, a pattern has been established. Continue with the pattern having each person toss the ball to the same person when it goes around again. Add more balls to the game challenging the group to handle the chaos.

- Have the class sit on a hard floor to participate in a lummi sticks activity. Demonstrate how to make certain rhythmical patterns using the lummi sticks. Have each student imitate the pattern and then take turns inventing a new pattern for the rest of the group to copy.

- Demonstrate how to use silk scarves for movement by juggling them and then tossing them to other members of the group. Vary the complexity of the juggling and the pattern of tossing.

- Demonstrate parachute activities using balls in the center of the parachute. Have group members run under the parachute. Create various patterns with the parachute while moving it up and down.

- Be sure to do a slow or cool-down activity at the end to get everyone's heart rate down to a normal speed.

2. Demonstrate to the students any other activities that you may have available, for example, use a large beachball to play volleyball, play basketball on a court, play badminton, or bowl using plastic pins.

3.a.–b. Have students put their ideas on flip charts for the entire class to see. To increase the creative challenge, assign students the same budget or equipment. Then see the different ideas that can be generated by different groups using the same amount of money or materials.

Follow-up

Refer to the chart below for the appropriate evaluative source most helpful in assuring that your students integrate the information from this exercise.

Application of Competencies (end of chapter 4 in CCOT)	Performance Skills (end of chapter 4 in CCOT)	Appendix (in CCOT)	Clinical Competency Checklist (appendix in IM)
X			

Leisure Planning

Study Questions–Key Terms/Readings

Use the chart below to find information addressing each study question. Look up the key terms in the sources given in the suggested readings column. Refer to the index, the table of contents (T.O.C.), or other locations as indicated.

Study Questions	Key Terms	Suggested Readings
1.	Leisure-time occupations, definition of play and leisure	Stein—index
2.	Leisure-time occupations, assumptions underlying leisure activities	Stein—index
3.	Leisure Skills	Early—T.O.C.
4.	Leisure Skills	Early—T.O.C.
5.	Leisure Skills	McCarthy—T.O.C.
6.	Leisure-time occupations, identifying client interest	Stein—index
	Leisure Assessments	Asher—T.O.C.
7.a.–g.	Leisure Skills	Early—T.O.C.
8.	Reflective	
9.	Reflective	Local phone book and newspaper

Activity–Teaching Strategies

1.a.–c. You may use a leisure assessment from Asher (1996) or one that you have selected from another source. Once the activities outlined in a–c are completed, ask the students to write a leisure goal for themselves. Students often think they should stop participating in all leisure activities once they are busy in an academic program. This is a good time to talk about "balance" in one's life and to explain that when a person is the most stressed, that is the time to care the most for oneself. Encourage students who are not participating in any leisure activities to write a goal concerning the specific activity and the amount of time they will participate in that activity. If students get stuck in the process, provide a brainstorming session having other peers offer suggestions. Plan a group leisure-time activity as a result of this discussion, such as an outing to a local zoo, a midmorning group game of volleyball, or an evening at the symphony.

2.a.–b. Assign students the identical case studies, changing only the cultural information of the client. See what differences were suggested in the activity choices. Discuss how one's culture can influence the leisure-time interests and choices of a client.

Follow-up

Refer to the chart below for the appropriate evaluative source most helpful in assuring that your students integrate the information from this exercise.

Application of Competencies (end of chapter 4 in CCOT)	Performance Skills (end of chapter 4 in CCOT)	Appendix (in CCOT)	Clinical Competency Checklist (appendix in IM)
X			

Time Management

Study Questions–Key Terms/Readings

Use the chart below to find information addressing each study question. Look up the key terms in the sources given in the suggested readings column. Refer to the index, the table of contents (T.O.C.), or other locations as indicated.

Study Questions	Key Terms	Suggested Readings
1.	Temporal adaptation	Mosey—index
2.	Time management, stress management and	Early—index
3.	Time management, anxiety disorders, and	Cara—index
4.	Time management, stress management and	Early—index
5.	Integrity in the Moment of Choice	Covey—T.O.C.
6.a.–f.	Temporal adaptation	Mosey—index
7.	Temporal adaptation, intervention process	Mosey—index
8.	Reflective	

Activity–Teaching Strategies

1. Completing the Idiosyncratic Activities Configuration is a very lengthy and time-consuming process. Give students ample warning so that they may work ahead. Alternatively, require only part of the configuration to be completed.

2. Discuss with students the use of this tool with clients who have multiple sclerosis, arthritis, or any illness requiring a careful look at the use of time in relationship to a person's values. The configuration can tell us much about our clients as we assist in planning their goals and treatment modalities.

3.a.–d. Use chart paper displayed around the room for students to complete their work. These charts will provide a visual display and a colorful description of personal differences. When thinking about how imbalance might be reflected, tell students to be realistic in the changes they feel are possible in their lives at the current time. When discussing how the activity may be used in treatment, have the students draw how the pie of life might look for a client who has a bipolar disorder in the manic phase and then what the pie would look like when that person is in the depressed phase. What would a pie of life look like for a client who has major depression and is unemployed receiving disability benefits.?

4.a.–b. Out of necessity and survival many students may be rather expert at time management especially if they are going to school and working, and have a family. Use this opportunity to allow those students to learn from each other about what works and what does not work. Everyone can benefit from learning about additional time management techniques or strategies!

Follow-up

Refer to the chart below for the appropriate evaluative source most helpful in assuring that your students integrate the information from this exercise.

Application of Competencies (end of chapter 4 in CCOT)	Performance Skills (end of chapter 4 in CCOT)	Appendix (in CCOT)	Clinical Competency Checklist (appendix in IM)
X			

Stress Management

Study Questions–Key Terms/Readings

Use the chart below to find information addressing each study question. Look up the key terms in the sources given in the suggested readings column. Refer to the index, the table of contents (T.O.C.), or other locations as indicated.

Study Questions	Key Terms	Suggested Readings
1.	Stress management program, program description	Cotrell—index
2.	Uniform Terminology	AOTA(latest edition)—index
3.	Stress and its relationship to mental illness, definition of	Stein—index
4.	Stress and its relationship to mental illness, causes of stress	Stein—index
5.	Stress, management of	Neidstadt—index
6.	Stress management program	Cotrell—index
7.a.–k.	Stress, management of	Neidstadt—index
8.	Reflective	
9.a.–d.	Coping Skills Assessment	Tubesing—T.O.C.
10.	Reflective	
11.	Reflective	
12.	Reflective	
13.	Stress Management Questionnaire	Stein—index
	Stress, management of	Neidstadt—index

Activity–Teaching Strategies

1. Use one of the stress inventories found in Tubesing and Tubesing (1994) or another of your choice. Use several different inventories and compare the instruments themselves as well as the results from each one.

2. This is an opportunity for the students to learn from each other about how to manage their stress. Some students may already successfully handle their course work as well their family and work responsibilities. However, some students may have difficulty handling the pressure, and this activity will serve as a resource for them to learn new ideas. Some students may also be in the habit of incorporating unhealthy methods to manage their stress such as drinking or using over the counter medications. Emphasize the need to keep stress management techniques from adding to poor health.

3. Consult Tubesing and Tubesing (1994) for many activity ideas on stress management. Participate in the activities yourself, demonstrating how fun they can be. Often it is a means of stress relief for students to see their instructor acting silly. Repeat a stress activity right before tests or whenever you determine the class is in need of such diversion. Encourage the class to request a stress reduction activity when they feel the need. A favorite activity is the "Shark Attack" described in Tubesing and Tubesing (1994).

4.a.–b. Instead of having the entire class plan activities for an acute-care adult setting, have them do other group settings, such as adolescence and chronic care. Discuss with the class how they as a group may want to focus on participating in stress reducing activities on occasion or on a regular basis. For a special treat show a video such as "Humor Your Stress" (L. Donnelley, 1996) Humor Potential, Boston MA. Incorporate ideas from the video in class.

Follow-up

Refer to the chart below for the appropriate evaluative source most helpful in assuring that your students integrate the information from this exercise.

Application of Competencies (end of chapter 4 in CCOT)	Performance Skills (end of chapter 4 in CCOT)	Appendix (in CCOT)	Clinical Competency Checklist (appendix in IM)
X	4D	B: Therapeutic Use of Self-Analysis	

Psychosocial Groups

Study Questions–Key Terms/Readings

Use the chart below to find information addressing each study question. Look up the key terms in the sources given in the suggested readings column. Refer to the index, the table of contents (T.O.C.), or other locations as indicated.

Study Questions	Key Terms	Suggested Readings
1.	Current Practice in Occupational Therapy	Howe–T.O.C.
2.	Current Practice in Occupational Therapy	Howe–T.O.C.
3.	Groups, advantages/limitations	Cara–index
4.	Group process, applying to psychosocial occupational therapy, establishing of group goals	Stein–index
5.	Activity groups, types	Stein–index
6.	Groups, leaders of	Cara–index
7.	Reflective	
8.	Group therapy, short-term psychiatric setting, flexibility	Cotrell–index
9.	Therapeutic groups	Neidstadt–index
10.a.–e.	Activity groups, developmental	Mosey–index
11.	Activity groups, developmental	Mosey–index

Activity–Teaching Strategies

1. Encourage students to use a variety of groups in order to incorporate the different interests of their clients. Discuss with the students the type and amount of space they will need to run the groups, as well as an estimate of the financial start-up costs of their proposed groups.

2. Use the group protocol outlined in Cole (1998) or another of your choice. Give the students a time limit in which to demonstrate their groups. Have students lead the groups during future sessions; this scheduling will allow students to bring supplies they will need.

Follow-up

Refer to the chart below for the appropriate evaluative source most helpful in assuring that your students integrate the information from this exercise.

Application of Competencies (end of chapter 4 in CCOT)	Performance Skills (end of chapter 4 in CCOT)	Appendix (in CCOT)	Clinical Competency Checklist (appendix in IM)
X	4C, 4F	B: Therapeutic Use of Self-Analysis	X

Intervention Planning

Study Questions–Key Terms/Readings

Use the chart below to find information addressing each study question. Look up the key terms in the sources given in the suggested readings column. Refer to the index, the table of contents (T.O.C.), or other locations as indicated.

Study Questions	Key Terms	Suggested Readings
1.	Standards of Practice for Occupational Therapy	AOTA(latest edition)–T.O.C.
2.	Standards of Practice for Occupational Therapy	AOTA(latest edition)–T.O.C.
3.	Intervention(s), interviewing to establish priorities for	Neidstadt–index
4.	Families, importance in health care	Neidstadt–index
5.	Motivation, intervention to build	Neidstadt–index
6.	Observation notes	Early–index
7.	Roles and Functions Papers: Occupational Therapy Roles	AOTA(latest edition)–T.O.C.
8.	Goals, in psychiatric rehabilitation	Early–index
9.	Responding to Symptoms and Behaviors	Early–T.O.C.
10.a.–e.	Human Occupation and Mental Health Throughout the Life Span	Early–T.O.C.
11.	Culture, occupational process and	Cara–index
12.	Craft activities, anxiety disorders and	Cara–index
13.	Craft activities, anxiety disorders and	Cara–index

Activity–Teaching Strategies

1,2,3. Supply OTA students with information for subparts a and c, and have the students complete subparts b, d, e, and f. If you are a clinical supervisor, have your OTA and OT students work together on this project. Assign the third case study to be completed individually by each student. Have students bring the completed case studies in for discussion.

4. Invite other faculty members or staff members from your facility to join in listening to the student's presentations.

5. Schedule a time to meet with students who are continuing to have difficulty with treatment planning. If there are several students who find themselves in this circumstance, assist them in forming a study group. Provide them with continued direction and practice.

Follow-up

Refer to the chart below for the appropriate evaluative source most helpful in assuring that your students integrate the information from this exercise.

Application of Competencies (end of chapter 4 in CCOT)	Performance Skills (end of chapter 4 in CCOT)	Appendix (in CCOT)	Clinical Competency Checklist (appendix in IM)
X	4A, 4G	B: Therapeutic Use of Self-Analysis	X

Psychosocial Health, Wellness and Prevention

Study Questions—Key Terms/Readings

Use the chart below to find information addressing each study question. Look up the key terms in the sources given in the suggested readings column. Refer to the index, the table of contents (T.O.C.), or other locations as indicated.

Study Questions	Key Terms	Suggested Readings
1.	Occupational therapy, historical developments	Bruce—index
2.	Substance abuse treatment, issues	Cara—index
3.a.	Substance abuse, definitions concerning	Cara—index
b.	Eating disorders causes, onset, and course of	Neidstadt—index
4.a.	Substance abuse, treatment, planning; Substance abuse, treatment, approaches	Cara—index
b.	Eating disorders	Neidstadt—index
5.	Reflective	Local newspaper and telephone book
6.	Reflective	
7.	Reflective	

Activity—Teaching Strategies

1. Have students bring index cards with them and put each agency's basic information on a card. Alternatively, have students enter the information into a computer database. Discuss the need to develop a resource file for all areas of practice. Keep your own file so that you may supplement the students' lists as well as add any new resources that have been identified by the students to your list.

2. Have students discuss whether there are barriers that would keep the client from accessing the suggested resources. Discuss what resources may be helpful to the client that are unavailable in your community.

3.a.–b. Prior to class have each student attend a group in the community that uses a twelve-step approach. Have the students share their experiences with the class. Invite a chemical dependency counselor to class to lead such a group for the students. There is a good chance that most of the class is affected in some way by substance abuse either personally or knowing someone who has an addiction, therefore, having students participate in a twelve-step group similar to Al-Anon would be appropriate. Invite an occupational therapy practitioner who works with substance abuse clients to lead or discuss the twelve-step method, sharing how knowledge of it will assist in treatment.

Follow-up

Refer to the chart below for the appropriate evaluative source most helpful in assuring that your students integrate the information from this exercise.

Application of Competencies (end of chapter 4 in CCOT)	Performance Skills (end of chapter 4 in CCOT)	Appendix (in CCOT)	Clinical Competency Checklist (appendix in IM)
X			

Section Four

Performance Skill 4A

Adding to Your Files

Add categories to the targeted areas as is appropriate for your students. Have students target activities for certain practice settings such as acute adult inpatient, adolescent outpatient substance abuse unit, chronic institutionalization, geriatric psychiatry, and so on. Have students find certain activities for certain diagnoses, such as schizophrenia, bipolar disorder, eating disorder, borderline personality disorder, and the like.

Performance Skill 4B

Interview

Consider asking a graduate of your program to volunteer to be the client for this interview, or ask students in your drama program to role-play for the client in the interview. (Taking part would allow them to practice their acting skills while helping you out.) Either give students information on the client ahead of time or when it is time for them to conduct their interview. Use a structured interview (appropriate for OTA students) or an open-ended interview (appropriate for OT students). Alternatively, have students generate and use their own interview questions. As a part of this assignment, ask students to hand in summaries of their interviews, as well as treatment plans listing suggested activities for intervention. If students perform poorly allow them to watch the videotape and critique their performance, writing down statements they wish they would have said or would not have said. Have them critique their nonverbal communication as well.

Performance Skill 4C

Planning a Group

Have students lead this group at their fieldwork site on approval of their fieldwork educator (practice setting). Have a clinician provide the situation to the students depicting a real-life situation with case studies. Have students work individually or together to complete this skill.

Performance Skill 4D

Group Activity

Each student will need to have time to lead a group activity that includes discussion. Divide the class into two groups and sit between the two so that you can grade two students at a time. This way each student will have more time to lead his or her group. To make this performance skill more challenging, assign antigroup roles to one or two members of the class in order to evaluate the leader's ability to deal with such behaviors in a therapeutic manner.

Performance Skill 4E

Teaching a Basic Life Task

Make sure students bring the resources they will need in order to teach the basic life task in a hands-on fashion. Encourage students to be creative in their teaching techniques. For example, duplicate the face of a money station machine using large cardboard pieces. Have students prepare and then lead this group at their field-work site on approval of their fieldwork educator (practice setting).

Performance Skill 4F — More Practice with Your Teaching

Assign each student a certain craft that you would like the class to learn or allow students to choose the craft they would like to teach. Select crafts that are frequently used in your community OT settings. Keep updated by periodically asking your clinical supervisors about most recent practices. Take advantage of the annual clinical educators meetings or your institution's advisory committee meetings to help keep you up-to-date.

Performance Skill 4G — Intervention Planning

Give this as an individual assignment. Provide OTA students with the problems and goals prior to working the treatment plan; have OT students complete the entire plan. Have students complete this assignment using any of the cases at the end of the section or any other of your choice.

References

Allen, C. K. (1990). Allen Cognitive Level (ACL) Screening test. Available from Allen Conferences, Inc.

Allen, C. K. n.d. Ribbon Cards. Available from Allen Conferences, Inc. Ormond Beach, FL.

Allen, C. K., C. A. Earhart, and T. Blue. 1992. *Occupational Therapy Treatment Goals for the Physically and Cognitively Disabled*. Rockville, MD: American Occupational Therapy Association.

Asher, I. E. 1996. *Occupational Therapy Assessment Tools: An Annotated Index*. 2d ed. Bethesda, MD: American Occupational Therapy Association.

Brayman, S. J., and T. Kirby. 1976. *Comprehensive Occupational Therapy Evaluation (COTE)*. *American Journal of Occupational Therapy*, 30(2): 94–100.

Bruce, M. A., and B. Borg. 1993. *Psychosocial Occupational Therapy: Frames of Reference for Intervention*. 2d ed. Thorofare, NJ: Slack.

Cara, E., and A. MacRae. 1998. *Psychosocial Occupational Therapy in Clinical Practice*. Albany: Delmar Publishers.

Christiansen, C. and C. Baum. eds. 1997. *Occupational Therapy: Enabling Function and Well-Being*. 2d ed. Thorofare, NJ: Slack.

Cole, M. B. 1998. *Group Dynamics in Occupational Therapy: The Theoretical Basis and Practice Application of Group Treatment*. 2d ed. Thorofare, NJ: Slack.

Cottrell, R. P. F. 1993. *Psychosocial Occupational Therapy: Proactive Approaches*. Bethesda, MD: American Occupational Therapy Association.

Covey, S. R., A. R. Merrill, and R. R. Merrill, 1994. *First Thing's First*. New York: Simon and Schuster.

Cynkin, S., and A. M. Robinson. 1990. *Occupational Therapy and Activities Health: Toward Health Through Activities*. Boston: Little, Brown.

Davis, C. M. 1998. *Patient Practitioner Interaction: An Experiential Manual for Developing the Art of Health Care*. 3rd ed. Thorofare, NJ: Slack.

Denton, P. L. 1987. *Psychiatric Occupational Therapy: A Workbook of Practical Skills*. Boston: Little, Brown.

Dynes, R. 1993. *Creative Games in Group Work*. Bichester, England: Winslow Press.

Earhart, C. A., C. K. Allen, and T. Blue. 1993. *Allen Diagnostic Manual: Instruction Manual*. Available from Allen Conferences, Inc., Ormond Beach, FL.

Early, M. B. 2000. *Mental Health Concepts and Techniques for the Occupational Therapy*

Assistant. 3rd ed. Philadelphia: Lippincott Williams & Wilkins.

Hemphill-Pearson, B. J. ed. 1999. *Assessments in Occupational Therapy Mental Health.* Thorofare, NJ: Slack.

Howe, M. C., and S. L. Schwartzberg. 1995. *A Functional Approach to Group Work in Occupational Therapy.* Philadelphia: J. B. Lippincott.

Korb-Khalsa, K. L., S. D. Azok, and E. A. Leutenberg. 1995. *S.E.A.L. + Plus.* Beechwood, OH: Wellness Reproductions.

McCarthy, K. 1993. *Activities of Daily Living: A Manual of Group Activities and Written Exercises.* Framingham, MA: Therapro.

Mosey, A. C. 1986. *Psychosocial Components of Occupational Therapy.* New York: Raven Press.

Neidstadt, M. E., and E. B. Crepeau. eds. 1998. *Willard and Spackman's Occupational Therapy.* 9th ed. Philadelphia: J. B. Lippincott.

Purtillo, R., and A. Haddad. 1996. *Health Professional and Patient Interaction.* 5th ed. Philadelphia: W. B. Saunders.

Rider, B. B., and S. J. Rider. 1999. *The Book of Activity Cards for Mental Health.* Kalamazo, MI: Authors.

Ross, M. 1997. *Integrative Group Therapy: Mobilizing Coping Abilities with the Five-Stage Group.* Bethesda, MD: American Occupational Therapy Association.

Stein, F., and S. K. Cutler. 1988. *Psychosocial Occupational Therapy: A Holistic Approach.* San Diego: Singular Publishing Group.

Thomson, L. K. 1992. *Kohlman Evaluation of Living Skills.* Bethesda, MD: American Occupational Therapy Association.

Tubesing, N. L., and D. A. Tubesing. 1994. *Structured Exercises in Stress Management: A Handbook for Trainers, Educators, and Group Leaders.* Vol. 1. Duluth, MN: Whole Person Associates.

University of Missouri. 1989. *Interference: A Simulation of the Symptoms, Systems, and Side Effects of Mental Illness.* Missouri: Author.

Williams, H. D., and J. Bloomer. 1987. *Bay Area Functional Performance Evaluation (BaFPE)* 2nd ed. Pequannock, NJ: Maddak.

Observation Skills

Study Questions—Key Terms/Readings

Use the chart below to find information addressing each study question. Look up the key terms in the sources given in the suggested readings column. Refer to the index, the table of contents (T.O.C.), or other locations as indicated.

Study Questions	Key Terms	Suggested Readings
1.	Observation	Early—index
2.	Asymmetry, evaluation in hemiplegia	Pedretti—index
3.	Hemiplegia, posture, typical adult	Pedretti—index
4.	Associated reactions	Pedretti—index
5.a.	Rheumatoid Arthritis	Pedretti—T.O.C.
b.	Cerebral Vascular Accident	Pedretti—T.O.C.
c.	Traumatic Brain Injury	Pedretti—T.O.C.
d.	Spinal Cord Injury	Pedretti—T.O.C.
e.	Hip Fractures and Total Hip Replacement	Pedretti—T.O.C.
f.	Oncology	Early—T.O.C.
g.	Pulmonary Disease	Early—T.O.C.
h.	Low Back Pain	Pedretti—T.O.C.
i.	Degenerative Diseases of the Central Nervous System	Pedretti—T.O.C.
j.	Burns and Burn Rehabilitation	Pedretti—T.O.C.
6.	Treatment, guiding	Trombly—index
7.	Observation, in treatment planning	Trombly—index
	Observation, reevaluation	Early—index
8.	Observation, in evaluation	Pedretti—index
9.	Evaluation	Pedretti—index

Activity—Teaching Strategies

1. Purchase a videotape or, with permission, videotape a client. Obtain a video-tape of a client who clearly has asymmetries and abnormal movement patterns (e.g., a client with a cerebral vascular accident). Role-play such a client as an alternative. After completing documentation of the observation process, repeat with a client having a different diagnosis.

Follow-up

Refer to the chart below for the appropriate evaluative source most helpful in assuring that your students integrate the information from this exercise.

Application of Competencies (end of chapter 5 in CCOT)	Performance Skills (end of chapter 5 in CCOT)	Appendix (in CCOT)	Clinical Competency Checklist (appendix in IM)
X			

Standardized Assessments

Study Questions—Key Terms/Readings

Use the chart below to find information addressing each study question. Look up the key terms in the sources given in the suggested readings column. Refer to the index, the table of contents (T.O.C.), or other locations as indicated.

Study Questions	Key Terms	Suggested Readings
1.	Clinical reasoning	Pedretti—index
2.	Standardized tests	Pedretti—index
3.a.–b.	Temporal context	Pedretti—index
4.a.–e.	Occupational Therapy Evaluation and Assessment of Physical Dysfunction	Pedretti—T.O.C.
5.	Standardized tests	Pedretti—index
6.	Standardized tests	Pedretti—index
7.a.–c.	Hand Injuries	Pedretti—T.O.C.
8.a.–d.	Hand Injuries	Pedretti—T.O.C.
9.	Hand Injuries	Pedretti—T.O.C.
10.	Reflective	

Activity—Teaching Strategies

1.a.–g. Spread tests around the room in stations and have students rotate between stations. Have students administer tests to peers in their class. Have students administer the tests to other students in lower-level classes as an introduction for those students to course content they will be learning later (see Chapter One, Exercise 16). Add other assessments to this activity that may be commonly used in your community.

2. Encourage students to spend time practicing their assessment skills after class hours. Critique their performances by completing the grid provided.

3. Have students practice administering the different assessments as part of this activity. Use the Competency Checklist A: Skill Assessment (Self/Instructor/Other) again as a means to evaluate students at a later date. Include their performances as part of the course grade.

Follow-up

Refer to the chart below for the appropriate evaluative source most helpful in assuring that your students integrate the information from this exercise.

Application of Competencies (end of chapter 5 in CCOT)	Performance Skills (end of chapter 5 in CCOT)	Appendix (in CCOT)	Clinical Competency Checklist (appendix in IM)
X			X

Muscle Testing

Study Questions–Key Terms/Readings

Use the chart below to find information addressing each study question. Look up the key terms in the sources given in the suggested readings column. Refer to the index, the table of contents (T.O.C.), or other locations as indicated.

Study Questions	Key Terms	Suggested Readings
1.	Evaluation of Muscle Strength	Pedretti—T.O.C.
2.	Functional muscle test	Pedretti—index
3.	Evaluation of Muscle Strength	Pedretti—T.O.C.
4.	Grading	Kendall—index
5.	Evaluation of Muscle Strength	Pedretti—T.O.C.
6.	Evaluation of Muscle Strength	Pedretti—T.O.C.
7.	Strength	Pedretti—index
8.	Endurance, strength and	Pedretti—index
9.	Substitution	Kendall—index
10.	Manual muscle test, procedure; Functional muscle test	Pedretti—index
11.	Manual muscle test, sequence	Pedretti—index
12.	Dynamometer	Pedretti—index
13.a.–f.	Functional muscle test	Pedretti—index

Activity–Teaching Strategies

1.–2. Have students give these strength tests to peers in their class as well as students in lower-level classes to give those students an introduction to testing, (See Chapter One, Exercise 16). Have students use the administration of these strength tests as a fund-raiser to make money while practicing, either as an independent fund-raiser or as part of an institution-wide fund-raiser. Have a contest to see who is the strongest in the class and/or facility/institution. Have age and gender brackets. Award simple prizes.

3. Demonstrate manual muscle testing procedures or have a clinician do so. Videotape the procedure. Put the videotape in a resource center for students to study at their convenience. Use a commercially obtained video or CD-ROM of manual muscle testing.

4. Demonstrate and practice one movement at a time or complete the test in total. Use a videotape of the procedure as described in #3 above. Have students follow along in one of their textbooks containing pictorial procedures.

Follow-up

Refer to the chart below for the appropriate evaluative source most helpful in assuring that your students integrate the information from this exercise.

Application of Competencies (end of chapter 5 in CCOT)	Performance Skills (end of chapter 5 in CCOT)	Appendix (in CCOT)	Clinical Competency Checklist (appendix in IM)
X			X

Vital Signs

Study Questions—Key Terms/Readings

Use the chart below to find information addressing each study question. Look up the key terms in the sources given in the suggested readings column. Refer to the index, the table of contents (T.O.C.), or other locations as indicated.

Study Questions	Key Terms	Suggested Readings
1.a.	Vital signs	Pierson—index
b.	Pulse, definition of	Pierson—index
c.	Respiration	Pierson—index
d.	Blood pressure	Pierson—index
e.	Tachycardia, definition of	Pierson—index
f.	Bradycardia, definition of	Pierson—index
g.	Hypotension, definition of	Pierson—index
h.	Hypertension, definition of	Pierson—index
i.	Dyspnea, definition of	Pierson—index
j.	Arrhythmia(s)	Pierson—index
k.	Bradypnea	Neidstadt—index
2.	Vital signs monitoring, in cardiopulmonary dysfunction	Neidstadt—index
3.	Pulse, sites for	Pierson—index
4.	Pulse, measurement of	Pierson—index
5 .	Pulse, abnormal	Pierson—index
6.	Pulse, normal range for; Blood pressure, normal range for	Pierson—index
7.	Blood pressure, measurement of	Pierson—index
8.	Respiration	Pierson—index
9.a.	Pulse, factors affecting	Pierson—index
b.	Blood pressure, factors affecting	Pierson—index
c.	Respiration, factors affecting	Pierson—index
10.	Vital signs	Rothstein—index
11.	Cardiovascular system dysfunction	Pedretti—index
12.	Cardiopulmonary resuscitation (CPR)	Pierson—index

Activity–Teaching Strategies

1. Demonstrate the vital-signs techniques. Have an experienced occupational therapist (OT) practitioner or other health professional demonstrate the techniques.

2. Have students practice on family members and personal friends. Have students practice their techniques on volunteers from within their facility or from the community. Have students practice these techniques at a health fair. Use this practice time as a promotion activity for OT. After obtaining an individual's vital signs, have students give them information on OT. Do this activity during National OT Month.

Follow-up

Refer to the chart below for the appropriate evaluative source most helpful in assuring that your students integrate the information from this exercise.

Application of Competencies (end of chapter 5 in CCOT)	Performance Skills (end of chapter 5 in CCOT)	Appendix (in CCOT)	Clinical Competency Checklist (appendix in IM)
X			X

Sensory Assessment and Reeducation

Study Questions–Key Terms/Readings

Use the chart below to find information addressing each study question. Look up the key terms in the sources given in the suggested readings column. Refer to the index, the table of contents (T.O.C.), or other locations as indicated.

Study Questions	Key Terms	Suggested Readings
1.	Sensation, dysfunction	Pedretti–index
2.	Sensation	Trombly–index
3.a.–g.	Sensation, tests	Pedretti–index
4.	Evaluation of Sensation	Trombly–T.O.C.
5.a.–e.	Sensation, treatment	Pedretti–index
6.a.–f.	Sensation, dysfunction; treatment	Pedretti–index

Activity–Teaching Strategies

1. Demonstrate sensory testing procedures for your students or videotape a clinician completing sensory testing. Have your host institution offer to videotape the clinician. Use a copy of the videotape for your class. Give a copy to the clinician to be used for his or her student program or training new therapists.

2. Acknowledge that students may find their partners have sensory deficits. Have students inquire of their partners whether or not an injury has been suffered or if awareness of the deficit is known. If students want a second opinion, have other students perform the same test on them.

3. The olfactory and gustatory sensation tests are infrequently performed, so not as much time should be spent here.

4. Demonstrate the effects of sensory deficits in an activity such as transferring from wheelchair to bed. Have each group practice performing the transfer while a student role-plays having the deficit.

5. Use the procedures from the game Battleship™ for this activity. Have the student being tested mark his or her sensory test form in several locations indicating where they will pretend to have sensory deficits. Have the student administering the test do so by trying to find the other student's assumed

deficits. Once the assessment is complete, have the two students compare forms to see if all the assumed deficits were found.

6. Several remedial treatment programs are described in Pedretti (1996), including those by individuals such as Dellon, Wynn Parry, Turner, and La Croix and Helman.

Follow-up

Refer to the chart below for the appropriate evaluative source most helpful in assuring that your students integrate the information from this exercise.

Application of Competencies (end of chapter 5 in CCOT)	Performance Skills (end of chapter 5 in CCOT)	Appendix (in CCOT)	Clinical Competency Checklist (appendix in IM)
X			X

Transfers and Positioning

Study Questions–Key Terms/Readings

Use the chart below to find information addressing each study question. Look up the key terms in the sources given in the suggested readings column. Refer to the index, the table of contents (T.O.C.), or other locations as indicated.

Study Questions	Key Terms	Suggested Readings
1.	Body mechanics, principles of	Pierson—index
2.	Transfers, assistance with	Trombly—index
3.	Transfers, types of	Pierson—index
4.a.	Sliding board transfer, to wheelchair	Pedretti—index
b.	Sliding board, sitting transfers with	Pierson—index
5.	Sliding board, sitting transfers with	Pierson—index
6.	Transfer(s), precautions for	Pierson—index
7.	Wheelchair Assessment and Transfers	Pedretti—T.O.C.
8.	Transfer(s), standing	Pierson—index
9.a.	Bed, positioning, for beginning level traumatic brain injury and for hemiplegic patient	Pedretti—index
b.	Positioning, in spinal cord injury	Trombly—index
10.a.–c.	Bed, positioning, for hemiplegic patient	Pedretti—index

Activity–Teaching Strategies

1. Have students complete activities pertaining to body mechanics in Exercise 41, if not already completed. Emphasize the importance of using correct body mechanics for ease of lifting as well as for safety to self and client.

2. Generate conditions for the discussion such as pain, obesity, body side neglect, pushing syndrome, cognitive deficits, spasticity, and communication deficits.

3. Demonstrate variations in correct positioning. Adhere to precautions to maintain the client's shoulder and hip integrity.

4. Demonstrate these techniques. Critique students on their use of correct procedure.

5.–6. On completion of this competency, have students do an inservice to other students at your host institution as a part of their course work. If you are in a clinical setting, have students instruct nursing students or other staff members, taking the opportunity to further master of this essential skill. Pairing with students in another department, such as nursing, can be an avenue of increasing interdisciplinary communication. A student who qualifies for accommodations set forth by the Americans with Disabilities Act (ADA) can demonstrate competence in verbally instructing transfers to individuals not yet familiar with these techniques.

Follow-up

Refer to the chart below for the appropriate evaluative source most helpful in assuring that your students integrate the information from this exercise.

Application of Competencies (end of chapter 5 in CCOT)	Performance Skills (end of chapter 5 in CCOT)	Appendix (in CCOT)	Clinical Competency Checklist (appendix in IM)
X			X

Range of Motion

Study Questions—Key Terms/Readings

Use the chart below to find information addressing each study question. Look up the key terms in the sources given in the suggested readings column. Refer to the index, the table of contents (T.O.C.), or other locations as indicated.

Study Questions	Key Terms	Suggested Readings
1.	Range of Motion (ROM)	Pedretti—index
2.	Active range of motion, definition	Trombly—index
3.	Passive range of motion, definition	Trombly—index
4.	Goniometers, in range of motion measurement	Trombly—index
5.	Evaluation of Joint Range of Motion	Pedretti—T.O.C.
6.	Evaluation of Joint Range of Motion	Pedretti—T.O.C.
7.	Evaluation of Joint Range of Motion	Pedretti—T.O.C.
8.	Evaluation of Joint Range of Motion	Pedretti—T.O.C.
9.	Range of motion, functional	Pedretti—index
10.	Range of motion, limitations	Pedretti—index
11.	Evaluation of Joint Range of Motion	Pedretti—T.O.C.
12.	Range of motion record, upper extremity, procedure	Daniels—index

Activity—Teaching Strategies

1. In your discussion, include at least the following principles: establish rapport with client, know normal range of each joint, know functional aspect of each movement, note any sounds (indicating possible complications) while extremity is moving, and move only in the range comfortable to the client unless otherwise specified. Additionally, include in your discussion at least the following precautions: respect pain, follow physician-ordered precautions, support the weight of the extremity if necessary, and avoid ranging a shoulder without simultaneously feeling for the integrity of the shoulder joint.

2. Demonstrate range of motion (ROM) movements and then allow students time to practice. Students should know these movements and their names by the end of this activity.

3. Demonstrate the complete ROM assessment procedure. Textbooks offering pictorial guidelines are often helpful as students are first learning measurement procedures. Allow students time to practice while you continue to in-

struct and assess their competency. Extra boxes are included on the grid for the students to continue their practice.

4. Encourage the students to be specific in the skills a person may not be able to perform. For example, an individual having only 90 degrees should flexion would be unable to comb his or her hair. Discuss compensatory techniques (using the other hand) and adaptive equipment (an angled hair brush) that may be used to increase independence.

5. Demonstrate proper technique for passive ROM procedures. Demonstrate retrograde massage if time permits.

6. When playing this advanced game of Simon Says, have students unable to assume the position and range be the next caller. Congratulate the winner or award the individual with a small prize.

7. Use this as part of the student's grade for the course. Have students include this as part of their portfolios.

Follow-up

Refer to the chart below for the appropriate evaluative source most helpful in assuring that your students integrate the information from this exercise.

Application of Competencies (end of chapter 5 in CCOT)	Performance Skills (end of chapter 5 in CCOT)	Appendix (in CCOT)	Clinical Competency Checklist (appendix in IM)
X			X

Activities of Daily Living

Study Questions–Key Terms/Readings

Use the chart below to find information addressing each study question. Look up the key terms in the sources given in the suggested readings column. Refer to the index, the table of contents (T.O.C.), or other locations as indicated.

Study Questions	Key Terms	Suggested Readings
1.	Activities of daily living, definition	Trombly–index
2.	Activities of daily living, definition	Trombly–index
3.	Common terminology used in occupational therapy	AOTA(latest edition)–other
4.	Activities of Daily Living	Pedretti–T.O.C.
5.	Activities of Daily Living	Pedretti–T.O.C.
6.	Activities of daily living, education	Trombly–index
7.a.–f.	Activities of daily living (ADL), recording results of	Pedretti–index
8.	Activities of daily living (ADL), training	Pedretti–index
9.	Activities of Daily Living	Pedretti–T.O.C.
10.a.–b.	Dressing activities, in hemiplegia	Pedretti–index
11.	Reflective	
12.	Evaluation of Activities of Daily Living (ADL) and Home Management	Neidstadt–T.O.C.
13.	The Meaning of Self-Care Occupations	Christiansen–T.O.C.

Activity–Teaching Strategies

1. Generate the different conditions from your discussion. Conditions may include, but are not limited to, the following: deficits in memory, sequencing, body scheme, praxis, and proprioception.

2. Obtain videos of clients with the identified diagnosis who have mastered these specified activities of daily living (ADL) skills. Such videos may be obtained from practitioners supervising fieldwork students who may use them as part of their student training program.

3. Discuss initial treatment and then gradation of these activities as the client improves. Instruct students to role-play realistic client deficits.

4. Have students put their information on flip charts and present this information to their classmates.

Follow-up

Refer to the chart below for the appropriate evaluative source most helpful in assuring that your students integrate the information from this exercise.

Application of Competencies (end of chapter 5 in CCOT)	Performance Skills (end of chapter 5 in CCOT)	Appendix (in CCOT)	Clinical Competency Checklist (appendix in IM)
X			X

Wheelchairs

Study Questions–Key Terms/Readings

Use the chart below to find information addressing each study question. Look up the key terms in the sources given in the suggested readings column. Refer to the index, the table of contents (T.O.C.), or other locations as indicated.

Study Questions	Key Terms	Suggested Readings
1.	Part II Evaluation and Prescription Principles and Practices	Trefler—T.O.C.
2.	Principles of Evaluation	Trefler—T.O.C.
3.	Assessment	Mayall—T.O.C.
4.a.–d.	Wheelchairs	Pedretti—index
	Wheelchairs, assessment team and	Angelo—index
5.	Wheelchairs, measurement procedure	Pedretti—index
	Wheelchair Features and Activities	Pierson—T.O.C.
6.	Wheelchair(s), fit of, back height and, confirmation of	Pierson—index
7.	New Moves	Scared Heart—video
8.a.–e.	Wheelchair, selection	Pedretti—index
9.	Safety Issues	Trefler—T.O.C.
10.	Wheelchair Assessment and Transfers	Pedretti—T.O.C.
11.a.–c.	Funding	Angelo—T.O.C.
12.	Wheelchairs, slection	Trombly—index
13.	Wheelchairs	Pedretti—index
	Principles of Evaluation	Trefler—T.O.C.

Activity–Teaching Strategies

1. Have a vendor from a Durable Medical Equipment (DME) supplier come to class to discuss the vendor's role in ordering wheelchairs for clients. Have that individual bring a variety of different types of wheelchairs for the students to use for this activity.

2. Liken this activity to what students will need to do when clients in a skilled nursing facility already have a chair but need adaptations to obtain correct positioning and alignment.

3. Have students seated on a mat table or similar firm surface while being measured. Make sure that students understand how to obtain the correct mea-

surement from the client as well as translate that measurement into the correct size of the wheelchair part needed.

4.a.–b. Have students practice their instructional techniques using the different wheelchair models available. Have students share feedback on the effectiveness of their instructional techniques with their partners.

Follow-up

Refer to the chart below for the appropriate evaluative source most helpful in assuring that your students integrate the information from this exercise.

Application of Competencies (end of chapter 5 in CCOT)	Performance Skills (end of chapter 5 in CCOT)	Appendix (in CCOT)	Clinical Competency Checklist (appendix in IM)
X			X

Cognitive Impairment

Study Questions–Key Terms/Readings

Use the chart below to find information addressing each study question. Look up the key terms in the sources given in the suggested readings column. Refer to the index, the table of contents (T.O.C.), or other locations as indicated.

Study Questions	Key Terms	Suggested Readings
1.	Cognition, definition	Trombly–index
2.	Executive functions	Zoltan–index
3.	Evaluation and Treatment of Cognitive Dysfunction	Pedretti–T.O.C.
4.	Cognition, deficits	Pedretti–index
5.a.–g.	Cognition, retraining	Pedretti–index
5.a.,b.,f.–k.	Theoretical Basis for Evaluation and Treatment	Zoltan–T.O.C.
6.	Attention	Zoltan–index
	Memory	Zoltan–index
	Initiation	Zoltan–index
	Awareness	Zoltan–index
	Organization	Zoltan–index
	Problem solving	Zoltan–index
	Mental flexibility	Zoltan–index
	Generalization	Zoltan–index
	Acalculia	Zoltan–index
7.	Ranchos Los Amigos Scale of Cognitive Functioning	Pedretti–index

Activity–Teaching Strategies

1. As students act out the terms, the true meaning of the words may not be apparent, for example, for mental flexibility, a student points to his head and then bends over backwards. If lack of understanding is apparent, be sure to discuss the correct meaning of the terms and clarify it with the class. Note, though, that students will be able to remember the term by recalling the humorous depiction.

2. Have students participate in the various cognitive activities you have provided (math worksheets, looking up numbers in a telephone book, etc.). Divide the class into groups and have each group analyze a specific cognitive

activity in more detail. Have the students problem-solve and think of other activities that could fulfill the same therapeutic purpose.

3. Students may put their case study presentations on flip charts and then present the same to the class. Highlight the safety precautions.

Follow-up

Refer to the chart below for the appropriate evaluative source most helpful in assuring that your students integrate the information from this exercise.

Application of Competencies (end of chapter 5 in CCOT)	Performance Skills (end of chapter 5 in CCOT)	Appendix (in CCOT)	Clinical Competency Checklist (appendix in IM)
X			X

Perceptual Impairments

Study Questions–Key Terms/Readings

Use the chart below to find information addressing each study question. Look up the key terms in the sources given in the suggested readings column. Refer to the index, the table of contents (T.O.C.), or other locations as indicated.

Study Questions	Key Terms	Suggested Readings
1.	Perception, definition	Trombly—index
2.	Factors That Influence the Patient's Vision, Perception, and Cognition	Zoltan—T.O.C.
3.a.–i.	Theoretical Basis for Evaluation and Treatment	Zoltan—T.O.C.
4.	Astereognosis	Pedretti—index
	Somatognosia	Zoltan—index
	Ideational apraxia	Zoltan—index
	Ideamotor apraxia	Zoltan—index
	Constructional apraxia	Zoltan—index
	Dressing apraxia	Zoltan—index
	Tactile agnosia	Zoltan—index
	Figure ground perception	Zoltan—index
	Homonymous hemianopsia	Pedretti—index
	Unilateral body neglect	Zoltan—index

Activity–Teaching Strategies

1. Discuss the meaning of each term after it has been guessed. For additional fun, have all groups send a designated "drawer" to the board at the same time for an "all play." This activity allows all teams to guess at the same time.

2. Use the materials listed and demonstrate any or all of the following suggested types of activities. Teach an individual with a perceptual deficit how to put on a shirt or pair of pants, brush his teeth or hair, and wash or shave his face. Use a weighted cuff to assist the individual in "feeling" his extremity as it moves thus improving body scheme. Use the colored tape to make an object stand out from its background or to direct the gaze of a person with hemianopsia to one side of a tray or table. Have an individual complete a figure ground worksheet to improve figure ground skills, or use a functional approach of engaging that individual in a cooking activity having her find the utensils in a cluttered utensil drawer. Have a client propel a wheelchair while working on improving her unilateral neglect. Use vibration to assist a client in improving his tactile

awareness and stereognosis abilities. On completion of these demonstrations, have students participate in the same activities and keep a journal about their experiences.

3. Have students share their treatment approaches with each other. Review the safety precautions that need to be followed for individuals with perceptual deficits.

Follow-up

Refer to the chart below for the appropriate evaluative source most helpful in assuring that your students integrate the information from this exercise.

Application of Competencies (end of chapter 5 in CCOT)	Performance Skills (end of chapter 5 in CCOT)	Appendix (in CCOT)	Clinical Competency Checklist (appendix in IM)
X			

Neurodevelopmental Treatment

Study Questions—Key Terms/Readings

Use the chart below to find information addressing each study question. Look up the key terms in the sources given in the suggested readings column. Refer to the index, the table of contents (T.O.C.), or other locations as indicated.

Study Questions	Key Terms	Suggested Readings
1.a.	Neurodevelopmental treatment (NDT); weight-bearing over affected side	Pedretti—index
b.	NDT, trunk rotation	Pedretti—index
c.	NDT, scapular protraction	Pedretti—index
d.	NDT, pelvis position	Pedretti—index
e.	NDT, slow, controlled movements	Pedretti—index
f.	NDT, positioning, proper	Pedretti—index
1.a.–f.	Neurodevelopmental (Bobath) Treatment	Trombly—T.O.C.
2.	NDT, therapeutic activity selection	Pedretti—index
3.	NDT, initiation	Pedretti—index
4.a.	Flaccidity, in hemiplegia	Pedretti—index
	Flaccidity, in stroke	Trombly—index
b.	Muscle tone, hypotonicity	Pedretti—index
c.	Spasticity, treatment, neurodevelopmental	Trombly—index
d.	Neglect, unilateral	Trombly—index
5.	Inhibition techniques, in neurodevelopmental treatment	Trombly—index
	Facilitation techniques, in neurodevelopmental treatment	Trombly—index
6.	NDT, patient evaluation	Pedretti—index

Activity—Teaching Strategies

1. Include in the discussion principles such as continual assessment, 24-hour approach, patterns of movement, abnormal tone, normal tone, not a dysfunctional side, amount of assistance to give, giving the correct amount of challenge, and quality motion.

2. Have students visualize a newborn baby coming home from the hospital. Describe how the infant eventually gets to a standing position.

3. Demonstrate the specified abnormal movement patterns for your class simulating someone who may have had a stroke. Freeze your movement patterns to

emphasize the difference between normal and impaired movement. Have a student demonstrate each designated movement pattern. Instruct the student to move as naturally as possible, asking that person to freeze at certain points so the movement can be observed closely. Videotape a client with a neurological impairment performing the movements specified. Stop and freeze the videotape to analyze each movement pattern.

4. Divide students into groups of two. Have one partner sit slumped forward with posterior pelvic tilt and give instructions to raise one arm above the head. Then have the student sit up straight and anteriorly tilt the pelvis while raising an arm. Have the other partner repeat the procedure. Discuss the importance of pelvic positioning as well as general postural alignment in upper-extremity mobility and functioning.

5. Create and make slides available with each designated technique for the students to study at the end of class. Videotape the students using the correct techniques and have the videotape available for review. Scan slides into a computer program for the students to use as a study guide. Introduce other techniques from NDT theory such as bilateral group activities, controlled one handed training, and so on.

6. In addition to case study #48, a variety of other case studies are applicable for this activity. Assist students in seeing how the principles of NDT can be used with clients of varied diagnoses.

7. Have students write their ideas on flip charts to assist in the discussion. Have the charts available for review.

Follow-up

Refer to the chart below for the appropriate evaluative source most helpful in assuring that your students integrate the information from this exercise.

Application of Competencies (end of chapter 5 in CCOT)	Performance Skills (end of chapter 5 in CCOT)	Appendix (in CCOT)	Clinical Competency Checklist (appendix in IM)
X			X

Proprioceptive Neuromuscular Facilitation

Study Questions–Key Terms/Readings

Use the chart below to find information addressing each study question. Look up the key terms in the sources given in the suggested readings column. Refer to the index, the table of contents (T.O.C.), or other locations as indicated.

Study Questions	Key Terms	Suggested Readings
1.a.–k.	Proprioceptive neuromuscular facilitation, effectiveness, principles	Trombly–index
2.a.–d.	The Proprioceptive Neuromuscular Facilitation Approach	Pedretti–T.O.C.
3.a.–f.	Proprioceptive neuromuscular facilitation, diagonal patterns in	Trombly–index
4.a.–e.	Proprioceptive neuromuscular facilitation (PNF), procedures	Pedretti–index
5.a.	Repeated contractions technique	Pedretti–index
b.	Rhythmical initiation	Pedretti–index
c.	Slow reversal	Pedretti–index
d.	Rhythmical stabilization	Pedretti–index
e.	Contract-relax	Pedretti–index
f.	Hold-relax	Pedretti–index
g.	Relaxation techniques	Pedretti–index
h.	Rhythmic rotation	Pedretti–index
6.	Proprioceptive neuromuscular facilitation, total patterns in	Trombly–index
7.	Proprioceptive neuromuscular facilitation, effectiveness, evaluation during	Trombly–index

Activity–Teaching Strategies

1. Have students use this time to learn the diagonal patterns. Briefly test their understanding and use of each diagonal pattern before having them learn the next one. Play a game of Simon Says to assess skills in a more enjoyable manner.

2. Review developmental postures that may be used in treatment to give students the needed background knowledge for this activity. Have students list their activities on a flip chart. Encourage students to use their creativity when selecting positions and activities for intervention.

Follow-up

Refer to the chart below for the appropriate evaluative source most helpful in assuring that your students integrate the information from this exercise.

Application of Competencies (end of chapter 5 in CCOT)	Performance Skills (end of chapter 5 in CCOT)	Appendix (in CCOT)	Clinical Competency Checklist (appendix in IM)
X			X

Spinal Cord Injury

Study Questions—Key Terms/Readings

Use the chart below to find information addressing each study question. Look up the key terms in the sources given in the suggested readings column. Refer to the index, the table of contents (T.O.C.), or other locations as indicated.

Study Questions	Key Terms	Suggested Readings
1.	Paraplegia	Pedretti—index
	Quadriplegia	Pedretti—index
	Tetraplegia, definition	Trombly—index
2.	Spinal cord injury, complete, incomplete	Trombly—index
3.	Spinal cord injury, treatment, precautions	Trombly—index
4.	Spinal cord injury; Occupational therapy protocol, recommended treatment techniques	Daniel—index
	Spinal cord injury; Occupational therapy protocol, paraplegia, recommended treatment techniques	Daniel—index
5.	Spinal cord injury, levels vs. treatment goals	Trombly—index
6.a.–c.	Spinal cord injury, psychological adjustment	Daniel—index
7.	Reflective	
8.	Occupational Performance: A Model for Practice in Physical Dysfunction	Pedretti—T.O.C.
9.a.–f.	Spinal cord injury; Occupational therapy protocol, initial evaluation	Daniel—index
	Spinal cord injury; Occupational therapy protocol, paraplegia, initial evaluation	Daniel—index
10.	Broadening the Construct of Independence	AOTA(1998)—T.O.C.
11.	Americans with Disabilities Act (ADA)	Pierson—index

Activity—Teaching Strategies

1.a. If no guests are available, select a level of spinal cord injury resulting in paraplegia and one resulting in tetraplegia. Divide the class into two groups. Have the groups role-play demonstrating how a person with this level of injury may complete the activities listed.

1.b. Have students reflect about the anticipated emotional adjustment to a spinal cord injury. Chances are someone in the group will have insight into this aspect from personal experience of knowing someone with such a disability.

2.a. Have the guest portray various emotions reflective of a newly injured client, including those of fear, anger, denial, and projection.

2.b. Have students discuss their feelings and the learning that occurred from participation in this activity.

3.a.–d. Assign different levels of injury to different students in your class. Have students present the same ADL and home management tasks to the entire class so that everyone's learning includes all the different spinal cord levels of lesion. Do likewise with the group treatment plan.

Follow-up

Refer to the chart below for the appropriate evaluative source most helpful in assuring that your students integrate the information from this exercise.

Application of Competencies (end of chapter 5 in CCOT)	Performance Skills (end of chapter 5 in CCOT)	Appendix (in CCOT)	Clinical Competency Checklist (appendix in IM)
X	5A		X

Home Management

Study Questions–Key Terms/Readings

Use the chart below to find information addressing each study question. Look up the key terms in the sources given in the suggested readings column. Refer to the index, the table of contents (T.O.C.), or other locations as indicated.

Study Questions	Key Terms	Suggested Readings
1.a.–f.	Uniform Terminology for Occupational Therapy (Third Edition)	AOTA(1998)
	Home management activities	Pedretti–index
	Ways of Living	Christiansen–entire book
a.	Home management activities	Pedretti–index
b.	Meal Preparation & Training	Klinger–entire book
c.	Shopping	Klinger–index
d.	Money management	Pedretti–index
	Money handling, with visual impairment	Trombly–index
e.	Safety in the Home	Klinger–T.O.C.
	Kitchen Planning, Storage, and Home Modifications	Klinger–T.O.C.
f.	Safety in the Home	Klinger–T.O.C.
2.	Self-Care/Home Management	Pedretti–T.O.C.

Activity–Teaching Strategies

1.a. When making plans for the meal, if the listed skills can be accomplished in the main dish alone, side dishes may not be necessary. However, students on a limited budget often appreciate the benefit of a "full meal."

1.b.–c. Have students assume the following disabilities:

Cerebral vascular accident (CVA). Have students simulate hemiparesis by propelling the wheelchair with one foot and wearing a resting hand splint to be reminded of the affected body side limitations. Putting on sunglasses with paper covering half of each lens will simulate hemianopsia. A client who is aphasic can be simulated by having a student be silent throughout the activity.

Arthritis. Have students hold tennis balls in their hands while performing all tasks. Putting plastic wrap over the lenses of sunglasses will simulate glaucoma. Have the students use a walker and follow toe-touch weight-bearing precautions as if a total hip replacement had been undergone.

Vision impairment. Have students use a blindfold throughout the activity.

Quadriplegia/Tetraplegia. Have students use a wheelchair as well as wear mittens when engaging in all tasks.

Offer suggestions throughout the meal preparation as necessary to assist the process. Have students assume the role of group leader responsible for several clients assuming the listed disabilities.

2. Encourage students to think of home management areas other than cooking for which to generate treatment activities.

Follow-up

Refer to the chart below for the appropriate evaluative source most helpful in assuring that your students integrate the information from this exercise.

Application of Competencies (end of chapter 5 in CCOT)	Performance Skills (end of chapter 5 in CCOT)	Appendix (in CCOT)	Clinical Competency Checklist (appendix in IM)
X		B: Analysis of Self	X

Assistive Technologies

Study Questions–Key Terms/Readings

Use the chart below to find information addressing each study question. Look up the key terms in the sources given in the suggested readings column. Refer to the index, the table of contents (T.O.C.), or other locations as indicated.

Study Questions	Key Terms	Suggested Readings
1.a.	Impairment, definition of	Cook–index
b.	Disabilities, definition of	Cook–index
c.	Handicap, definition of	Cook–index
d.	Assistive technologies, definition of	Cook–index
e.	Rehabilitative technology, definition of	Cook–index
f.	Introduction and Overview	Cook–T.O.C.
g.	Introduction and Overview	Cook–T.O.C.
h.	Soft technologies	Cook–index
i.	Assistive technologies, hard technology components of	Cook–index
j.	Assistive technologies, appliances versus tools and	Cook–index
k.	Tools versus appliances	Cook–index
l.	Prosthetic device	Cook–index
m.	Minimal assistive technologies	Cook–index
n.	Maximal assistive technologies	Cook–index
o.	General-purpose assistive technologies	Cook–index
p.	Specific-purpose assistive technologies	Cook–index
q.	Commercial assistive technologies	Cook–index
r.	Custom assistive technologies	Cook–index
2.a.–l.	Glossary of Microcomputer Terminology and Other Suggested Resources	Cromwell–T.O.C.
3.	The Technology Toolbox	Alliance for Techology Access–T.O.C.
	The Activities: General-Purpose Extrinsic Enablers	Cook–T.O.C.
	The Activities: Performance Areas	Cook–T.O.C.
	Assistive technology devices and systems, modifications	Trombly–index
4.a.–d.	Recent Legislation Affecting the Application of Assistive Technologies	Cook–T.O.C.
5.	RESNA	Cook–index

Study Questions	Key Terms	Suggested Readings
6.	Helpful Resources and References	Alliance for Techology Access—T.O.C.
7.	Overview of Service Delivery in Assistive Technology	Cook—T.O.C.
8.	Assistive Technology in Occupational Therapy	Neidstadt—T.O.C.
9.a.–f.	The Technology Toolbox	The Alliance—T.O.C.
10.	Assistive technology	AOTA(latest edition)—other

Activity–Teaching Strategies

1. Have students use assistive devices to run these programs. Visit a hospital or community-based facility where computer programs are used as part of the occupational therapy (OT) intervention provided.

2. Obtain information on environmental control units from a local vendor or OT practitioner who specializes in this area. Visit a site where residents use environmental control devices. Discuss occupational therapy's role in linking clients with the appropriate assistive technology.

3. Encourage students to keep cost in mind as they make computer software recommendations and selections for their clients. An ideal "wish list" may be generated with items then prioritized according to need and cost.

4. Students may complete this activity outside of class as homework. If the activity is completed in class, make arrangements to have telephone and computer access available for all. The awarding of any small prize (can of soda, pen or pencil with the host institution's name, coupon for a discount at the bookstore or cafeteria of the host institution) will most likely be appreciated.

4.b.–d. Assign these activities as homework to be completed outside of class to allow for a more comprehensive search. Encourage students to record funding sources, Internet sites, and support groups obtained by other students. Suggest that these be kept as future resources in the clinic.

4.e.–f. Initiate a class discussion on the Americans with Disabilities Act (ADA) as well as on the other information obtained in this exercise.

Follow-up

Refer to the chart below for the appropriate evaluative source most helpful in assuring that your students integrate the information from this exercise.

Application of Competencies (end of chapter 5 in CCOT)	Performance Skills (end of chapter 5 in CCOT)	Appendix (in CCOT)	Clinical Competency Checklist (appendix in IM)
X	5B		X

Therapeutic Adaptations

Study Questions–Key Terms/Readings

Use the chart below to find information addressing each study question. Look up the key terms in the sources given in the suggested readings column. Refer to the index, the table of contents (T.O.C.), or other locations as indicated.

Study Questions	Key Terms	Suggested Readings
1.	Activity/activities, adapting	Pedretti—index
2.a.–c.	Activity/activities, adapting	Pedretti—index
d.–e.	Self-Care Strategies, for Persons with Movement Disorders	Christiansen—T.O.C.
f.	Managing Self-Care in Adults with Upper-Extremity Amputations	Christiansen—T.O.C.
	Stroke, compensation techniques and contextual training	Christiansen—index
3.	Assistive Technology Evaluation Process	Neidstadt—index
	Adaptive strategies, recommendation of	Christiansen—index
	Assistive technology devices, selection of	Christiansen—index
4.	Assistive technology consumer empowerment and devices	Christiansen—index
5.	Therapeutic Partnerships: Caregiving in the Home Setting	Christiansen—T.O.C.
6.a.	Grooming aids	Christiansen—index
b.	Oral hygiene	Christiansen—index
c.	Self-Care Strategies for Persons with Rheumatic Diseases	Christiansen—T.O.C.
d.	Toileting	Christiansen—index
e.	Sexuality, hygiene and	Pedretti—index
f.	Dressing	Christiansen—index
g.	Feeding, eating, adaptive equipment for	Christiansen—index
h.	Medication, medi-planner; medication organizer	Arthritis Foundation—index
i.	Health maintenance	Christiansen—index
j.	Recreation and Leisure	Arthritis Foundation—T.O.C.
k.	Communication, assistive technology devices for	Christiansen—index
l.	Functional mobility	Christiansen—index
m.	Community transport	Christiansen—index
n.	Emergency response	Christiansen—index
o.	Issues of Sexuality with Physical Dysfunction	Pedretti—T.O.C.
p.	Home management skills, clothing care as	Christiansen—index
q.	Home management skills, meal preparation and cleanup and	Christiansen—index

Study Questions	Key Terms	Suggested Readings
r.	Shopping	Christiansen—index
s.	Money management	Christiansen—index
t.	Household maintenance, assistive technology devices for	Christiansen—index
u.	Safety rails/grab bars	Arthritis Foundation—index
v.	Child care	Arthritis Foundation—index
w.	Self-care Strategies for Children with Developmental Disabilities	Christiansen—T.O.C.
x.	Employment and Vocational Aids	Arthritis Foundation—T.O.C.
y.	Recreation and Leisure	Arthritis Foundation—T.O.C.

Activity–Teaching Strategies

1.a.–b. Have multiple copies of catalogues from several different companies available for this exercise. Emphasize the need to keep updated as new adaptive equipment is made available. Encourage students to write down the name of the supplier of the catalogue as well as the phone number of the company. Suggest that students join the mailing list of the company if they would like to receive personal copies of the catalogue at home.

2.a.–b. Promote enthusiastic creativity by offering a prize for the most original or unique solution.

3. When completing this activity in class, have telephones available for each group or pair of students. To save time and ensure that all vendors are represented, have a previously compiled list of suggested vendors available. Assign this activity to be completed outside of class.

Follow-up

Refer to the chart below for the appropriate evaluative source most helpful in assuring that your students integrate the information from this exercise.

Application of Competencies (end of chapter 5 in CCOT)	Performance Skills (end of chapter 5 in CCOT)	Appendix (in CCOT)	Clinical Competency Checklist (appendix in IM)
X	5D		X

Medical Equipment in Client Care

Study Questions—Key Terms/Readings

Use the chart below to find information addressing each study question. Look up the key terms in the sources given in the suggested readings column. Refer to the index, the table of contents (T.O.C.), or other locations as indicated.

Study Questions	Key Terms	Suggested Readings
1.a.–p.	Special Equipment and Patient Care Environments	Pierson—T.O.C.
2.	Cardiac Dysfunction	Pedretti—T.O.C.
	Intensive care unit, occupational therapy, for traumatic brain injury	Pedretti—index
3.	Special Equipment and Patient Care Environments	Pierson—T.O.C.
4.a.–c.	Infection Control and Safety Issues in the Clinic	Early—T.O.C.

Activity—Teaching Strategies

1.a.–b. If it is not possible to visit a unit, have a guest who works in intensive care speak with your class. Assist your guest by offering to visit his or her facility to take slide pictures or videotape the pieces of medical equipment to assist in that person's presentation. Discuss the students' impressions, fears, and concerns about the different pieces of equipment.

2.a.–b. Prior to beginning this activity, discuss the use of cotreatment in an intensive care setting. Have the guest speaker remain for this activity and offer feedback to the students on the ideas they generate. Ask the guest speaker to bring a case study from his or her facility to use for this activity.

Follow-up

Refer to the chart below for the appropriate evaluative source most helpful in assuring that your students integrate the information from this exercise.

Application of Competencies (end of chapter 5 in CCOT)	Performance Skills (end of chapter 5 in CCOT)	Appendix (in CCOT)	Clinical Competency Checklist (appendix in IM)
X			

Home Health

Study Questions–Key Terms/Readings

Use the chart below to find information addressing each study question. Look up the key terms in the sources given in the suggested readings column. Refer to the index, the table of contents (T.O.C.), or other locations as indicated.

Study Questions	Key Terms	Suggested Readings
1.	The Home Health Industry: Definitions, History, and Types of Service Delivery	Commission on Practice—T.O.C.
2.	Clinical Considerations for the Treatment of Patients with Physical Disabilities in Home Health	Commission on Practice—T.O.C.
	Mental Health Services in the Home Health Setting; Special Considerations	Commission on Practice—T.O.C.
	Home health	Lewis—index
3.	Home health	Lewis—index
4.	Home health	Lewis—index
	The Home Health Industry: Definitions, History, and Types of Service Delivery	Commission on Practice—T.O.C.
5.	Teamwork, Personnel Issues, and Supervision in the Home Health Setting	Commission on Practice—T.O.C.
6.	Teamwork, Personnel Issues, and Supervision in the Home Health Setting	Commission on Practice—T.O.C.
7.	The Home Health Industry	Commission on Practice—T.O.C.

Activity–Teaching Strategies

1.a.–i. Discuss with the students the many diverse home health environments in which they may find themselves working. Supply students with specific descriptions of environments ranging from a home in Beverly Hills to a one-room efficiency on top of a gas station. Discuss personal safety measures needed when working in a home health setting, including the use of cellular phones, personal alarm devices, and cotreatments, as well as a general awareness of unsafe situations. Discuss the pros and cons of being a home health practitioner. Emphasize the appropriateness of this practice area for an experienced practitioner. Help students understand that due to the complex issues and level of independence needed, practicing in a home health setting is not recommended for new graduates. Discuss how OTA supervision is handled in a home health setting.

Follow-up

Refer to the chart below for the appropriate evaluative source most helpful in assuring that your students integrate the information from this exercise.

Application of Competencies (end of chapter 5 in CCOT)	Performance Skills (end of chapter 5 in CCOT)	Appendix (in CCOT)	Clinical Competency Checklist (appendix in IM)
X			

Work Hardening

Study Questions–Key Terms/Readings

Use the chart below to find information addressing each study question. Look up the key terms in the sources given in the suggested readings column. Refer to the index, the table of contents (T.O.C.), or other locations as indicated.

Study Questions	Key Terms	Suggested Readings
1.a.	Work practice	Jacobs–index
b.	Work hardening	Neidstadt–index
c.	Work conditioning	Neidstadt–index
2.	History of Work Practice in Occupational Therapy	Jacobs–T.O.C.
3.	Work hardening, process	Pedretti–index
4.	Work hardening	Pedretti–index
	Work practice	Jacobs–index
5.	Work-hardening team	Neidstadt–index
6.a.–c.	Appendix: Guidelines for Work Hardening Programs	Jacobs–T.O.C.
7.	Work hardening, milieu	Pedretti–index
8.	Work Assessments	Jacobs–T.O.C.
9.	Job simulation	Jacobs–index
	Simulated job work samples	Jacobs–index
10.	Job site analysis	Neidstadt–index
	Job analysis	Jacobs–index
11.	Work hardening	Neidstadt–index
12.	Work practice information	AOTA(latest edition)–other
13.	Ergonomic standards information	www.osha.gov
14.	Industrial rehabilitation	Internet

Activity–Teaching Strategies

1.a.–e. If a site visit is not possible, viewing a videotape or slides works well for this practice area. On-site or pictorial support is helpful due to the unique nature of the work hardening environments. Discuss the psychological aspects of working with clients in this setting. Additionally, discuss the role of the occupational therapy practitioner in industrial rehabilitation settings. Include the ramification of the implementation of the recent ergonomic standards.

2. If using a guest speaker, align the length and the hours of the program to that of the specific site described.

Follow-up

Refer to the chart below for the appropriate evaluative source most helpful in assuring that your students integrate the information from this exercise.

Application of Competencies (end of chapter 5 in CCOT)	Performance Skills (end of chapter 5 in CCOT)	Appendix (in CCOT)	Clinical Competency Checklist (appendix in IM)
X	5F		X

Pain Management

Study Questions–Key Terms/Readings

Use the chart below to find information addressing each study question. Look up the key terms in the sources given in the suggested readings column. Refer to the index, the table of contents (T.O.C.), or other locations as indicated.

Study Questions	Key Terms	Suggested Readings
1.	Pain, chronic	Neidstadt–index
	Pain, acute vs. chronic	Jacobs–index
2.	Pain, definition	Trombly–index
3.	Pain, chronic, psychosocial characteristics of	Jacobs–index
4.	Pain behavior	Jacobs–index
5.	Pain, management of	Neidstadt–index
6.	Pain, management of	Neidstadt–index
7.	Work Programs for Adults with Neurophysiologic Problems	Jacobs–T.O.C.
8.	Pain, evaluation of	Neidstadt–index
	Pain rating scales and questionnaires	Jacobs–index
9.	Pain rating scales and questionnaires	Jacobs–index
10.	Pain and Basic Stress Management	Catalano–T.O.C.
11.	Dealing with Others	Catalano–T.O.C.

Activity–Teaching Strategies

1.a.–b. Rather than having students generate their own, supply case studies for them. Have students write a proposal for a new outpatient pain management program to be presented and considered by a hospital administrator. Have students determine the cost associated with this proposal.

Follow-up

Refer to the chart below for the appropriate evaluative source most helpful in assuring that your students integrate the information from this exercise.

Application of Competencies (end of chapter 5 in CCOT)	Performance Skills (end of chapter 5 in CCOT)	Appendix (in CCOT)	Clinical Competency Checklist (appendix in IM)
X			

Splinting

Study Questions–Key Terms/Readings

Use the chart below to find information addressing each study question. Look up the key terms in the sources given in the suggested readings column. Refer to the index, the table of contents (T.O.C.), or other locations as indicated.

Study Questions	Key Terms	Suggested Readings
1.	Splints/splinting	Pedretti–index
2.	Introduction to Splinting	Coppard–T.O.C.
	Down: 1. Memory 2. Splint 3. Bonding 4. Dynamic	
	Across: 1. Elasticity 2. Orthosis 3. Dynamic 4. Drapability	
3.	Upper extremity splinting, purpose of	Neidstadt–index
4.	Upper extremity splinting, biomechanics and	Neidstadt–index
5.	Precautions, in clinical examination	Coppard–index
6.a.	Properties of Thermoplastic Splinting Materials	Rehabilitation Division, Smith and Nephew–T.O.C.
b.	Objectives and Principles of Static Splinting	Rehabilitation Division, Smith and Nephew–T.O.C.
c.	Objectives and Principles of Static Splinting	Rehabilitation Division, Smith and Nephew–T.O.C.
7.	Upper extremity splinting, functional vs. antideformity position and	Neidstadt–index

Activity–Teaching Strategies

1. Encourage students to practice identifying arches and creases of the hand using the CD-ROM, Splinting Made Easy: Just Add Water (Rehabilitation Division, Smith and Nephew, 1997).

2. Supply static as well as dynamic hand splints for students. Have splints available for the lower extremities, trunk, and neck.

3. Have students form each piece of splinting material in the web space of their thumbs. Ask students to identify the type of material with which they were most successful in molding and with which they felt most comfortable.

4.a.–d. Grade completed splints as part of the student's grade for the course. Provide students with recommendations on needed adjustments prior to such grading. Allow final splint adjustments and include peer feedback after wearing the splint in the final grading process. Discuss the student's experience wearing the splint, specifically including how it affected daily living skills.

Follow-up

Refer to the chart below for the appropriate evaluative source most helpful in assuring that your students integrate the information from this exercise.

Application of Competencies (end of chapter 5 in CCOT)	Performance Skills (end of chapter 5 in CCOT)	Appendix (in CCOT)	Clinical Competency Checklist (appendix in IM)
X		B: Analysis of Self	X

Upper Extremity Amputations and Prosthetics

Study Questions–Key Terms/Readings

Use the chart below to find information addressing each study question. Look up the key terms in the sources given in the suggested readings column. Refer to the index, the table of contents (T.O.C.), or other locations as indicated.

Study Questions	Key Terms	Suggested Readings
1.	Amputation (upper extremity)	Trombly–index
2.a.–c.	Amputation, upper extremity, levels	Pedretti–index
3.	Amputation and Prosthetics	Trombly–T.O.C.
4.	Amputation, upper extremity, special considerations/problems	Pedretti–index
5.	Amputation, upper extremity, psychological adjustments	Pedretti–index
6.a.–b.	Terminal device, for body-powered prostheses	Pedretti–index
7.a.–e.	Amputation, upper extremity, functional training with	Pedretti–index

Activity–Teaching Strategies

1.a.–i. Invite a prosthetist to be a guest speaker. Plan a field trip to a site where prosthetic devices are fabricated and fitted to see the variety of devices available.

2. Complete this activity in the lab or at a site where prosthetic devices are fabricated. Have students list the muscles necessary to operate each prosthetic device.

Follow-up

Refer to the chart below for the appropriate evaluative source most helpful in assuring that your students integrate the information from this exercise.

Application of Competencies (end of chapter 5 in CCOT)	Performance Skills (end of chapter 5 in CCOT)	Appendix (in CCOT)	Clinical Competency Checklist (appendix in IM)
X			

Hand Therapy and Physical Agent Modalities

Study Questions–Key Terms/Readings

Use the chart below to find information addressing each study question. Look up the key terms in the sources given in the suggested readings column. Refer to the index, the table of contents (T.O.C.), or other locations as indicated.

Study Questions	Key Terms	Suggested Readings
1.	Impairments of Hand Function	Trombly—T.O.C.
2.a.	Reflex sympathetic dystrophy, upper extremity, hand	Trombly—index
b.	Scar, remodeling, in hand injury treatment	Pedretti—index
c.	Flexor tendons, repair	Trombly—index
d.	Edema	Pedretti—index
e.	Hand, nerves, postoperative management of	Pedretti—index
3.	Paraffin baths	Pedretti—index
	Hot packs	Pedretti—index
	Cryotherapy	Pedretti—index
	Whirlpool baths	Trombly—index
	Electrical stimulation	Trombly—index
	Fluidotherapy	Trombly—index
	Transcutaneous electrical nerve stimulation description	Pedretti—index
4.	Physical Agent Modalities	Trombly—T.O.C.
5.	Physical agent modalities	AOTA(latest edition)—index
6.	Physical agent modalities	State Licensure Law

Activity–Teaching Strategies

1.a. Schedule a field site visit in a hand therapy clinic or a hospital-based site where clients with hand injuries are seen. Have students interact with the following physical agent modalities: paraffin, fluidotherapy, electrical stimulation, heat packs, ice, and whirlpool. Arrange to have an occupational therapist as well as a client at the clinic talk to the students during their visit.

1.b. Discuss the impact a hand injury has on a person's use of hands, engagement in occupation, and overall sense of well-being.

2. Have a member of the staff at the hand center provide a case study for the students. Encourage students to plan their interventions for the individual in the case study while still at the hand clinic using the modalities and activities available there. Have students present their plans to the staff and solicit feedback on the same.

Follow-up

Refer to the chart below for the appropriate evaluative source most helpful in assuring that your students integrate the information from this exercise.

Application of Competencies (end of chapter 5 in CCOT)	Performance Skills (end of chapter 5 in CCOT)	Appendix (in CCOT)	Clinical Competency Checklist (appendix in IM)
X			

Intervention Planning

Study Questions–Key Terms/Readings

Use the chart below to find information addressing each study question. Look up the key terms in the sources given in the suggested readings column. Refer to the index, the table of contents (T.O.C.), or other locations as indicated.

Study Questions	Key Terms	Suggested Readings
1.a.	Occupational performance model, treatment continuum in	Pedretti–index
b.	Enabling activities	Pedretti–index
c.	Purposeful activity (occupation)	Pedretti–index
d.	Occupational performance model, treatment approaches and	Pedretti–index
2.	Exercise, therapeutic	Pedretti–index
3.	Exercise, therapeutic, purposes	Pedretti–index
4.	Exercise, therapeutic, prerequisites	Pedretti–index
5.a.	Exercise, therapeutic, for cardiovascular fitness	Pedretti–index
b.	Exercise, therapeutic, for range of motion	Pedretti–index
c.	Exercise, therapeutic, for coordination improvement	Pedretti–index
d.	Exercise, therapeutic, for muscle strength	Pedretti–index
e.	Exercise, therapeutic, isotonic active	Pedretti–index
f.	Exercise, therapeutic, isometric	Pedretti–index
6.	Exercise, therapeutic, classification	Pedretti–index
7.	Activity/activities selection	Pedretti–index
	Activity selection	Trombly–index
8.	Activity selection	Trombly–index
9.	Activity/activities, selection	Pedretti–index
10.	Exercise, therapeutic	Pedretti–index
11.	The Psychosocial Core of Occupational Therapy	AOTA(1998)–T.O.C.
12.	Client Centered Occupational Therapy	Law–T.O.C.
13.	Implementation, client centered occupational therapy services	Law–index
14.	Motivation, engagement and harnessing	Law–index

Activity–Teaching Strategies

1. Make this into a game having the most creative answer awarded a small prize. Have the class determine this by popular vote. Alternatively, have students

base their activity/occupation selections on different case studies. Have students share their selection of activities/occupations with their classmates before revealing the particulars of their case study. Have the other class members determine, from the activities/occupations alone, what the client's needs, roles, interests, culture, gender, diagnosis, might be. Challenge students to closely align their activity/occupation choices so the rationale is clearly seen.

2. Have small groups of students role play a treatment session they might convene with the client identified in the assigned case study. Have groups occur simultaneously moving between each group providing feedback on their interactions during the treatment session.

3. Come dressed to class imitating Regis Philbin wearing a shirt and tie of the the same color or imitating his current fashion choices. Add stage lights to complete the game ambiance. Keep track of scores and award the winner(s) practitioner-related prizes e.g., goniometer, pencil grip, tape measure, pen, therapathy™. Videotaping this game may be reviewed with humor upon students future graduation.

Follow-up

Refer to the chart below for the appropriate evaluative source most helpful in assuring that your students integrate the information from this exercise.

Application of Competencies (end of chapter 5 in CCOT)	Performance Skills (end of chapter 5 in CCOT)	Appendix (in CCOT)	Clinical Competency Checklist (appendix in IM)
X	5C, 5E		X

Section 5

Performance Skill 5A   ## Disability Simulation

Determine the disability to be assumed for the student or allow the student to choose. For instance, if you want them all to experience being in a wheelchair, specify whether they should simulate tetraplegia, paraplegia, or hemiplegia. Contact a local vendor to see if students might be permitted to borrow equipment for this assignment. Or allow students to simulate disabilities such as arthritis, amputation, or blindness.

Performance Skill 5B   ## Fabrication of Adaptive Device

Have students share their equipment with the class. Take pictures of the adaptive devices and have students put them in their portfolios. Encourage students to enter their adaptive device in the competition held by Maddak© or another rehabilitation equipment distributor at the annual American National Occupational Therapy Association Conference.

Performance Skill 5C   ## Adding to Your Files

Add performance or component areas to this list as you see the need. After completion of the activity or issuing of a grade, have the files containing the activity suggestions available for students to review the work of their peers. Have students share files by copying favorites from each other in order to expand their own files.

Performance Skill 5D   ## Activity Adaptation

Use the ideas suggested in 5B for this activity as well.

Performance Skill 5F   ## Intervention Planning

In this era of managed care, give this as an in-class assignment, thereby simulating the little time available to actually plan a client's treatment. Vary the length and the number of treatment sessions for which the student needs to develop a treatment plan.

Performance Skill 5F   ## Nontraditional Interventions

Use the nontraditional Intervention Peer Evaluation Form to assist you in calculating students' grades. Keep information from the presentations on file for future students to use as a reference.

References

Alliance for Technology Access. 1994. *Complete Resources for People with Disabilities: A Guide to Exploring Today's Assistive Technology.* Alameda, CA: Hunter House.

American Guidance Service. 1969. *Pennsylvania Bi-Manual Test.* Circle Pines, MN: Author.

American Occupational Therapy Association. 1998. *Reference Manual of the Official Documents of the American Occupational Therapy Association.* Bethesda, MD: Author.

American Occupational Therapy Association. latest edition. *Reference Manual of the Official Documents of the American Occupational Therapy Association.* Bethesda, MD: Author.

Americans with Disabilities Act of 1996. (PL101-336), 42 U.S.C., 12101, Federal Register, vol. 56:144, 35543–35591.

Angelo, J. 1997. *Assistive Technology for Rehabilitation Therapists.* Philadelphia: F. A. Davis.

Arthritis Foundation. 1988. *Guide to Independent Living for People with Arthritis.* Atlanta, GA: Author.

Catalano, E. M. 1987. *The Chronic Pain Control Workbook: A Step-by-Step Guide for Coping with and Overcoming Your Pain.* Oakland, CA: New Harbinger Publications.

Christiansen, C., ed. 2000. *Ways of Living: Self-Care Strategies for Special Needs.* 2nd ed. Rockville, MD: American Occupational therapy Association.

Colarusso, R. P., D. D. Hammill, and L. Merceir. 1995. *Motor-Free Visual Perception Test,* Rev. Novato, CA: Academic Therapy Publications.

Commission on Practice Home Health Task Force. 1995. *Guidelines for Occupational Therapy Practice in Home Health.* Bethesda, MD: Author.

Cook, A. M., and S. M. Hussey. 1995. *Assistive Technologies: Principles and Practice.* Boston: Mosby.

Coppard, B. M., and H. L. Lohman. 1996. *Introduction to Splinting: A Critical-Thinking and Problem-Solving Approach.* St. Louis, MO: Mosby.

Cromwell, F. S. 1986. *Computer Applications in Occupational Therapy.* New York: Haworth Press.

Daniel, M. S., and L. R. Strickland. 1992. *Occupational Therapy Protocol Management in Adult Physical Dysfunction.* Gaithersburg, MD: Aspen Publishers.

Daniels, L., and C. Worthington. 1986. *Muscle Testing: Techniques of Manual Examination.* 5th ed. Philadelphia: W. B. Saunders.

Early, M. B. 1998. *Physical Dysfunction Practice Skills for the Occupational Therapy Assistant.* St. Louis: Mosby.

Jacobs, K. 1991. *Work-Related Programs and Assessments.* 2d ed. Boston: Little, Brown.

Jebsen, R. H., N. Taylor, R. B. Trieschmann, M. J. Trotter, and L. A. Howard. 1996. "An Objective and Standardized Test of Hand Function." *Archives of Physical Medicine and Rehabilitation* (June): 311–319.

Kendall, F. P., E. K. McCreary, and P. G. Provance. 1993. *Muscles: Testing and Function.* 4th ed. Baltimore, MD: Williams & Wilkins.

Klinger, J. L. 1997. *Meal Preparation and Training: The Health Care Professional's Guide.* Thorofare, NJ: Slack.

Law, M. ed. 1998. *Client-centered occupational therapy.* Thorofare, NJ: Slack.

Lewis, S. C. 1989. *Elder Care in Occupational Therapy.* Thorofare, NJ: Slack.

Mathiowetz, V., K. Weber, N. Kashman, and G. Volland. 1985. Nine Hole Peg Test of Fine Motor Coordination. Bolingbrook, IL: Sammons Preston.

Mayall, J. K., and G. Desharnais. 1990. *Positioning in a Wheelchair: A Guide for Professional Care Givers of the Disabled Adult.* Thorofare, NJ: Slack.

Neidstadt, M. E., and E. B. Crepeau, eds. 1998. *Willard and Spackman's Occupational Therapy.* 9th ed. Philadelphia: Lippincott.

Occupational Safety and Health Administration: web site: http://www.osha.gov.

Pedretti, L. W. 1996. *Occupational Therapy: Practice Skills for Physical Dysfunction.* 4th ed. St. Louis, MO: Mosby.

Pierson, F. M. 1999. *Principles and Techniques of Patient Care.* Philadelphia: W. B. Saunders.

Ramsammy, H., and P. Brand. *Hand Volumeter.* Idyllwild, CA: Volumeters Unlimited.

Rothstein, J. M., S. H. Roy, and S. L. Wolf. 1998. *The Rehabilitation Specialist's Handbook.* Philadelphia: F. A. Davis.

Rehabilitation Division, Smith and Nephew. 1998. *Splinting Made Easy: Just Add Water.* Germantown, WI: Author.

Sacred Heart General Hospital Oregon Rehabilitation Center. 1987. *New Moves: Wheelchair Skills Video Series.* Programs 1 to 4. Eugene, OR: Author.

Sanford, J. A., R. J. Browne, and A. Turner. 1985–95. *Captain's Log: Cognitive Training System.* Richmond, VA: Braintrain.

Tiffin, J. 1960. *Purdue Pegboard.* Lafayette, IN: Lafayette Instrument.

Trefler, E., D. A. Hobson, S. J. Taylor, L. C. Monahan, and C. G. Shaw. 1993. *Seating and Mobility for Persons with Physical Disabilities.* San Antonio, TX: Therapy Skill Builders.

Trombly, C. A. 1995. *Occupational Therapy for Physical Dysfunction.* 4th ed. Baltimore, MD: Williams & Wilkins.

University of Minnesota Employment Stabilization Research Institute. 1993. *Minnesota Rate of Manipulation Test.* Circle Pines, MN: American Guidance Service.

Zoltan, B. 1996. *Vision, Perception, and Cognition: A Manual for the Evaluation and Treatment of the Neurologically Impaired Adult.* 3d ed. Thorofare, NJ: Slack.

Getting in Touch

Study Questions–Key Terms/Readings

Use the chart below to find information addressing each study question. Look up the key terms in the sources given in the suggested readings column. Refer to the index, the table of contents (T.O.C.), or other locations as indicated.

Study Questions	Key Terms	Suggested Readings
1.a.	Demographics	Lewis—index
b.	Minorities and aging	Lewis—index
c.	Cognition and the Aging Adult	Larson—T.O.C.
d.	Cognition and the Aging Adult	Larson—T.O.C.
e.	Demographics	Lewis—index
2.	Reflective	
3.	Demographics of the aging population, community-based practices and	Larson—index
4.	Cultural environment, aging and culture	Larson—index
5.a.	Social Security Act and amendments	Larson—index
b.	Supplemental Security Income	Lewis—index
c.	Older Americans Act	Lewis—index
		Larson—T.O.C.
d.	National Institute on Aging	Lewis—index
e.	Keeping Current with Government Programming	Larson—T.O.C.
f.	Keeping Current with Government Programming	Larson—T.O.C.
6.a.	Activity theory of maturation	Larson—index
b.	Disengagement theory of maturation	Larson—index
c.	Erickson, Erik, personality theory of maturation	Larson—index
d.	Peck, Robert, personality theory of maturation	Larson—index
e.	Kohlberg, L.	Lewis—index
7.	Long term care	AOTA(latest edition)—other

Activity–Teaching Strategies

1.a.–c. Assume the role of game overall director (g.o.d.) as indicated in the instructions of the game. The goal of this game is to have the students experience some of the injustices that elderly people encounter as a result of inaccurate perceptions. Accomplish the goal by becoming more controlling and insulting as the game progresses. Students will usually start out having a good time but after a while the mood will change if you are doing your job and becoming more difficult as the game progresses. Use your colleagues or other interdisciplinary faculty members to be co-leaders for each area of living. Reciprocate the favor and assist other interdisciplinary faculty in playing this game with their students.

2.a.–e., 3. In this activity you are helping the students to get in touch with the emotional aspects of the elderly population. It will help if you read this poem and essay in an empathetic manner or have an elderly person read it. Have your tissues ready.

Follow-up

Refer to the chart below for the appropriate evaluative source most helpful in assuring that your students integrate the information from this exercise.

Application of Competencies (end of chapter 6 in CCOT)	Performance Skills (end of chapter 6 in CCOT)	Appendix (in CCOT)	Clinical Competency Checklist (appendix in IM)
X			

Evaluation in Geriatrics

Study Questions—Key Terms/Readings

Use the chart below to find information addressing each study question. Look up the key terms in the sources given in the suggested readings column. Refer to the index, the table of contents (T.O.C.), or other locations as indicated.

Study Questions	Key Terms	Suggested Readings
1.a.	Introduction to In-Home Assessments of Older Adults	Emlet—T.O.C.
b.	Accessibility and Safety	Emlet—T.O.C.
c.	Assessing Activities of Daily Living	Emlet—T.O.C.
d.	Basic Mobility Needs	Emlet—T.O.C.
e.	Physical Systems Assessment	Emlet—T.O.C.
f.	Medication Management and the Elderly	Emlet—T.O.C.
g.	Assessing Nutritional Needs	Emlet—T.O.C.
h.	Assessing Social Function, Support, and Socioeconomic Status	Emlet—T.O.C.
i.	Assessing Disturbances in Mood, Thought, Memory	Emlet—T.O.C.
j.	Assessing Disturbances in Mood, Thought, Memory	Emlet—T.O.C.
k.	The Informal Caregiver	Emlet—T.O.C.
2.	Interview, guidelines	Emlet—index
3.a.–c.	Kielhofner, G.	Lewis—index
4.	Occupational Performance History Interview	Asher—index
5.a.–c.	Assessment of Occupational Functioning	Watts—T.O.C.

Activity—Teaching Strategies

1.a. Students may locate and make arrangements for their own community volunteers or you may make the arrangements for them. Either way the learning experience will be enhanced if the volunteer who is a typical and healthy elderly person is not an immediate family member. The student will then have a real-life opportunity to establish rapport and gain information from an individual with whom they are not yet comfortable or familiar. To make arrangements for your students, contact a facility (nursing home, community center, etc.) a few weeks prior to completing this activity. Locate a setting that may have residents of diverse cultures or from cultures unique to your class. Some facilities may select the residents for your students to interview; other facilities may post a sign-up sheet for the residents to indicate their interest in participating.

Have several extra volunteer residents on stand-by for any cancellations by other residents. At the time of the interviews, stay at the facility with the students to be available for questions and assistance. Be sure your students accurately explain to their volunteers the purpose of this interview. They will be practicing their interviewing skill and assessment administration on a typical adult, not conducting a formal assessment on an individual with suspected dysfunction.

1.b. Plan ahead for potential problems with the individual's attention span, possible memory lapse, or scheduling conflicts.

1.c.–e. Students need to practice administering the "Set Test" (Issacs and Kinnie, 1973) and "Mini Mental State" (Folstein, Folstein, and Meugn, 1975) prior to the interview. They will also need to familiarize themselves with the "Paracheck Geriatric Rating Scale" (Paracheck, 1986). For additional information on occupational performance interviewing methods, consult Kielhofner's *A Model of Human Occupation: Theory and Application* (Baltimore: Williams & Wilkens, 1995).

1.f. Overlap of activities into the different performance areas may occur. Define the boundaries of the three different areas (self-care, work, play/leisure) ahead of time.

1.g.–j. Discuss with your class insights obtained through this experience about the cultural differences, balance of the OT performance areas, and strengths and weakness of the individual whom they interviewed. Have students critique their own performances as a part of this discussion. Assure students that it is not uncommon to administer an assessment with minor errors or to fail to gain certain information when first learning how to give an assessment. Emphasize the modifications and changes students need to make when administering this interview and these screening tools the next time.

1.k.–l. Assist students in critiquing themselves by giving very specific suggestions for improvements.

Follow-up

Refer to the chart below for the appropriate evaluative source most helpful in assuring that your students integrate the information from this exercise.

Application of Competencies (end of chapter 6 in CCOT)	Performance Skills (end of chapter 6 in CCOT)	Appendix (in CCOT)	Clinical Competency Checklist (appendix in IM)
X		B: Therapeutic Use of Self-Analysis	X

Safety and Fall Prevention

Study Questions–Key Terms/Readings

Use the chart below to find information addressing each study question. Look up the key terms in the sources given in the suggested readings column. Refer to the index, the table of contents (T.O.C.), or other locations as indicated.

Study Questions	Key Terms	Suggested Readings
1.	Accessibility and Safety	Emlet–T.O.C.
2.	Emergency planning	Larson–index
	Accessibility and Safety	Emlet–T.O.C.
3.	Prevention of Falls in the Elderly	Larson–T.O.C.
4.a.–b.	Prevention of Falls in the Elderly	Larson–T.O.C.
5.a.–c.	Prevention of Falls in the Elderly	Larson–T.O.C.
6.a.–e.	SPLAT assessment for falls	Larson–index
7.	Fall prevention information	www.bu.edu/roybal
8.	National Institute on Aging, Age Page	Emlet–index
9.	Falls Interview Schedule	Larson–index
	Safety, environmental assessment	Emlet–index
	Environmental Checklists	Larson–index
10.	Accessibility and Safety	Emlet–T.O.C.
11.	Accessibility and Safety	Emlet–T.O.C.

Activity–Teaching Strategies

1.a. Students may locate a community facility where their fall and safety in-service presentation may be made, or you may make the arrangements for them. This exercise could easily be a service learning project. It could also be a promotional or educational activity to highlight OT month. Videotape the students during their practice presentations in class so that they may critique their own performances.

1.b. This assessment can be used as part of a student's grade. Your assessment as an instructor can be added and weighted heavier than the students' input.

1.c. Inevitably editing, reediting, and revising will be a part of the student's planning a presentation. Facilitate the student's understanding that these activities are always a part of the writing and planning process.

2.a.–b. Have students use case study #54 and generate a possible realistic floor plan for this client based on homes they have themselves visited. Grid paper may be used. The exit plan can be indicated with arrows. The available support system telephone numbers or medical alert systems in your community can be obtained from the yellow pages of the telephone book. Discussing different options from the same case study will help students see that there is usually more than one right answer.

Follow-up

Refer to the chart below for the appropriate evaluative source most helpful in assuring that your students integrate the information from this exercise.

Application of Competencies (end of chapter 6 in CCOT)	Performance Skills (end of chapter 6 in CCOT)	Appendix (in CCOT)	Clinical Competency Checklist (appendix in IM)
X	6D		X

Adapting Occupations and Environment

Study Questions–Key Terms/Readings

Use the chart below to find information addressing each study question. Look up the key terms in the sources given in the suggested readings column. Refer to the index, the table of contents (T.O.C.), or other locations as indicated.

Study Questions	Key Terms	Suggested Readings
1.	Aging: Theoretical Considerations and Bio-Physical Realities	Lewis—T.O.C.
2.	Aging: Theoretical Considerations and Bio-Physical Realities	Lewis—T.O.C.
	Universal precaution(s)	Pierson—index
3.a.	Visual intervention	Lewis—index
b.	Auditory interventions	Lewis—index
c.	Mobility	Lewis—index
d.	Environmental needs/concerns	Lewis—index
e.	Memory	Lewis—index
4.	Negotiability	Christiansen—index
5.	Environmental needs/concerns	Lewis—index
6.	Issues and Aging	Lewis—T.O.C.
7.	Caregivers	Lewis—index

Activity–Teaching Strategies

1. There are many videos available on this topic. Have videos available to the students in the resource center for additional study.

2. You may have the students choose their own activities or you may use an activity calendar from a local nursing home to provide ideas.

2.b. Compare and contrast a variety of living environments, for example, hospital, group home, skilled nursing facility, retirement community, and own home.

3. You may use the same case study for each group and change the living environment for the same case study. Discuss how the living environment change influenced the group's recommendations for adaptations.

Follow-up

Refer to the chart below for the appropriate evaluative source most helpful in assuring that your students integrate the information from this exercise.

Application of Competencies (end of chapter 6 in CCOT)	Performance Skills (end of chapter 6 in CCOT)	Appendix (in CCOT)	Clinical Competency Checklist (appendix in IM)
X	6C		X

Joint Protection, Energy Conservation and Work Simplification

Study Questions–Key Terms/Readings

Use the chart below to find information addressing each study question. Look up the key terms in the sources given in the suggested readings column. Refer to the index, the table of contents (T.O.C.), or other locations as indicated.

Study Questions	Key Terms	Suggested Readings
1.	Joint Protection and Energy-Conservation Instruction	Melvin–T.O.C.
	Energy conservation	Lewis–index
	Work simplification/efficiency	Lewis–index
	Joint Protection and Energy-Conservation Instruction	Melvin–T.O.C.
2.a.	Reflective	
b.	Rheumatoid Arthritis	Melvin–T.O.C.
3.	Overview of Therapy for Joint Disease	Melvin–T.O.C.
	Energy conservation for cardiopulmonary dysfunction	Neidstadt–index
4.a.–c.	Joint Protection and Energy Conservation Instruction	Melvin–T.O.C.

Activity–Teaching Strategies

1. Have adaptive equipment available for students to use as props. Additional Hollywood-type props may be helpful, such as microphones, hats, ties, and wigs. Videotape the info-mercials. Students may enjoy reviewing the videotape during one of the last classes of the year or at graduation functions at the end of their program of study.

2. The scenarios may be written or typed at the top of 8½-by-11-inch paper prior to meeting with your class. Have a simple prize for the winner or distribute the "Creative Student Award."

Follow-up

Refer to the chart below for the appropriate evaluative source most helpful in assuring that your students integrate the information from this exercise.

Application of Competencies (end of chapter 6 in CCOT)	Performance Skills (end of chapter 6 in CCOT)	Appendix (in CCOT)	Clinical Competency Checklist (appendix in IM)
X			

Joint Replacement

Study Questions–Key Terms/Readings

Use the chart below to find information addressing each study question. Look up the key terms in the sources given in the suggested readings column. Refer to the index, the table of contents (T.O.C.), or other locations as indicated.

Study Questions	Key Terms	Suggested Readings
1.	Hip Surgery	Melvin–T.O.C.
	Knee Surgery	Melvin–T.O.C.
	Precautions for you	Platt(1992a; 1992b)–other
2.	Knee Surgery	Melvin–T.O.C.
	Hip Surgery	Melvin–T.O.C.
3.	See individual subheadings	Platt(1992a; 1992b)–other
4.	Hip Surgery	Melvin–T.O.C.
	Knee Surgery	Melvin–T.O.C.

Activity–Teaching Strategies

1. Demonstrate a treatment session using the adapted equipment or use a videotape of an actual treatment session. Discuss the factors influencing the intervention (diagnosis, insurance, functional ability, living arrangements, etc.) with an individual having a THR.

2.a.–b. Assign the three case studies (#56, #57, #58) to different sets of student partners.

Follow-up

Refer to the chart below for the appropriate evaluative source most helpful in assuring that your students integrate the information from this exercise.

Application of Competencies (end of chapter 6 in CCOT)	Performance Skills (end of chapter 6 in CCOT)	Appendix (in CCOT)	Clinical Competency Checklist (appendix in IM)
X			

Remotivation and Reality Orientation

Study Questions—Key Terms/Readings

Use the chart below to find information addressing each study question. Look up the key terms in the sources given in the suggested readings column. Refer to the index, the table of contents (T.O.C.), or other locations as indicated.

Study Questions	Key Terms	Suggested Readings
1.	Remotivation therapy	Lewis—index
2.	Remotivation therapy	Lewis—index
3.	Remotivation therapy	Lewis—index
4.a.–e.	Remotivation therapy	Lewis—index
5.	Reality orientation	Lewis—index
6.	Reality orientation	Lewis—index
7.	Reality orientation	Lewis—index
8.	Reality orientation	Lewis—index
9.	Therapeutic Techniques	Miller—T.O.C.
10.	Memory, assessment	Emlet—index

Activity—Teaching Strategies

1.a. You may decide to give the students more specifics regarding the population and facility; for example, number of clients, ages, gender, level of care, environment, and diagnoses.

1.b. These group sessions will detail what is to happen in the group. The description part may include suggested verbatim directions and questions for the introduction, activity, and discussion. Bring items from home for this activity and make advance preparations.

2. Based on an remotivation as described by Miller, Peckham, Peckham (1995), a possible activity to use is bread making (students will enjoy eating the finished product). To set a climate of acceptance, a general welcoming and comments regarding the weather or current events would be appropriate. A pictorial cookbook, photograph of bread, or local newspaper article on bread will create a bridge to reality. Examining and manipulating the actual items used to make the breads, as well as eating it, and asking thought provoking questions

will help explore the world in which they live. Exploring the work of the world can be done by discussing the production, manufacturing, and distribution of bread both past and present, locally or regionally. A climate of acceptance brings closure to the group by summarizing the discussion and thanking members for their participation.

3.a.–b. Use the items the students have brought with them as idea generators. As students develop their themes, they may want to include additional items. Creativity will abound. Discuss benefits of planning in groups and using props to brainstorm. Emphasize the use of simplicity when deciding themes and activities. Have students lead the groups.

Follow-up

Refer to the chart below for the appropriate evaluative source most helpful in assuring that your students integrate the information from this exercise.

Application of Competencies (end of chapter 6 in CCOT)	Performance Skills (end of chapter 6 in CCOT)	Appendix (in CCOT)	Clinical Competency Checklist (appendix in IM)
X			

Dementia

Study Questions–Key Terms/Readings

Use the chart below to find information addressing each study question. Look up the key terms in the sources given in the suggested readings column. Refer to the index, the table of contents (T.O.C.), or other locations as indicated.

Study Questions	Key Terms	Suggested Readings
1.	Dementia, introduction to	Holden—index
2.	Dementia, classification of	Larson—index
3.	Dementia, introduction to	Holden—index
4.	Mental disorders, patterns of development	Larson—index
5.	The Basic Approach to the Person with Dementia	Holden—T.O.C.
6.	Sensory deprivation, stimulation and activity	Holden—index
7.	Alzheimer's disease and other dementias	AOTA(latest edition)—other
8.	Behavior modification, problem behaviour	Holden—index
9.	Global deterioration scale	Lewis—index
10.	Validation therapy	Miller—index
11.	Validation theory	Lewis—index
12.a.–f.	Attitude therapy	Lewis—index
13.	Respite care	Lewis—index
14.	Group Work with People with Dementia	Holden—T.O.C.
15.	101 Ideas for Group Sessions	Holden—T.O.C.

Activity–Teaching Strategies

1. There are no right or wrong answers for this activity, although some may be more appropriate than others. Have the students decide which of their classmates' responses would be most helpful when working with actual clients.

2.a.–f. For additional learning, have students locate community agencies that may be of assistance to this client. Telephone inquiries made by the students may also reveal housing appropriate for this client.

Follow-up

Refer to the chart below for the appropriate evaluative source most helpful in assuring that your students integrate the information from this exercise.

Application of Competencies (end of chapter 6 in CCOT)	Performance Skills (end of chapter 6 in CCOT)	Appendix (in CCOT)	Clinical Competency Checklist (appendix in IM)
X			

Sensory Stimulation

Study Questions–Key Terms/Readings

Use the chart below to find information addressing each study question. Look up the key terms in the sources given in the suggested readings column. Refer to the index, the table of contents (T.O.C.), or other locations as indicated.

Study Questions	Key Terms	Suggested Readings
1.	Sensory deprivation, stimulation and activity	Holden—index
2.	Aging: Theoretical Considerations and Bio-Physical realities	Lewis—T.O.C.
3.	Sensory stimulation	Miller—index
4.	Sensory stimulation	Miller—index
5.	Sensory stimulation groups	Miller—index
6.	Sensory stimulation, one-to-one sensory stimulation	Miller—index
7.a.–e.	Sensory training	Lewis—index
8.	Sensory training	Lewis—index
9.a.	Introduction	Ross—T.O.C.
b.	Introduction	Ross—T.O.C.
c.	Introduction	Ross—T.O.C.
d.	Chapters 1–5	Ross—T.O.C.
10.a.–f.	Reflective	

Activity–Teaching Strategies

1.a. To help students visualize the functioning level of clients who are suited for this type of intervention, demonstrate some of the behaviors clients may exhibit and explain them in detail, or have the students visit a nursing home to observe a sensory stimulation group.

1.b. Emphasize the wide variety of options available for such a group. Feedback given can be written or verbal.

2. As part of your discussion, have students compare the differences between a sensory stimulation group and Ross's (1997) five-stage group. Emphasize Ross's strong theoretical and neurological base. Capitalize on students' creative ideas.

Follow-up

Refer to the chart below for the appropriate evaluative source most helpful in assuring that your students integrate the information from this exercise.

Application of Competencies (end of chapter 6 in CCOT)	Performance Skills (end of chapter 6 in CCOT)	Appendix (in CCOT)	Clinical Competency Checklist (appendix in IM)
X	6C		X

Eating, Feeding and Dysphagia

Study Questions–Key Terms/Readings

Use the chart below to find information addressing each study question. Look up the key terms in the sources given in the suggested readings column. Refer to the index, the table of contents (T.O.C.), or other locations as indicated.

Study Questions	Key Terms	Suggested Readings
1.a.–c.	Dysphagia, cause, description	Reed—index
2.a.–d.	Dysphagia	Lewis—index
3.	Dysphagia	Lewis—index
4.	Dysphagia	Lewis—index
5.	Eating	Lewis—index
6.	Eating, assistance with	Larson—index
7.	Dining room programs	Lewis—index
8.	Dining room programs	Lewis—index
9.	Dysphagia	Lewis—index
10.	Eating dysfunction	AOTA(latest edition)—other
11.	Dysphagia, assessment	Reed—index
12.	Videofluoroscopy	Early—index
13.	Eating dysfunction	AOTA(latest edition)—other
14.	Feeding and eating	AOTA(latest editon)—other

Activity–Teaching Strategies

1. If possible, have students observe an actual videofluoroscopy performed at a local hospital.

2. If your students have not completed the Exercise 44 in Chapter Three, you may have them do so at this time. Experiencing feeding difficulties themselves will encourage students to be more empathetic towards their future clients.

3. Take this activity one step further. Have students write up a proposal to start such a group in a nursing home. Include rationale, frame of reference, goals of the program, projected cost, and a time schedule.

Follow-up

Refer to the chart below for the appropriate evaluative source most helpful in assuring that your students integrate the information from this exercise.

Application of Competencies (end of chapter 6 in CCOT)	Performance Skills (end of chapter 6 in CCOT)	Appendix (in CCOT)	Clinical Competency Checklist (appendix in IM)
X			

Leisure Time

Study Questions–Key Terms/Readings

Use the chart below to find information addressing each study question. Look up the key terms in the sources given in the suggested readings column. Refer to the index, the table of contents (T.O.C.), or other locations as indicated.

Study Questions	Key Terms	Suggested Readings
1.	Leisure activities, definition	Larson—index
2.	Leisure time	Lewis—index
3.	Reflective	
4.	Leisure activities, occupational therapist role in	Larson—index
5.a.	Stress	Lewis—index
b.	Stress, sense of control and	Larson—index
6.	Wellness Model	Miller—index
7.	Volunteer participation	AOTA(latest edition)—other
8.a.–j.	Issues and Aging	Lewis—T.O.C.
9.	Leisure Assessments	Asher—T.O.C.

Activity–Teaching Strategies

1. Follow along with the videotape as your students participate in the "Range of Motion (ROM) Dance" (St. Mary's Hospital Medical Center and Board of Regents of the University of Wisconsin System, 1984). Emphasize the importance of slow, gentle movements. If students find such movements helpful to them personally, they may benefit from participating in tai chi classes in their community for their own health and well-being.

2. Have students set the environment for relaxation: dim lights, use blankets and pillows, close the door, cover the windows, close the blinds, and so on.

3.a.–b. Students may share their ideas verbally with the class.

4. Have resources available for the students to browse through once their lists are complete. Resources such as activity calendars or announcements of events, activities, and groups may be available from retirement communities and senior citizen centers. You may also ask students to bring some of these items from their local neighborhood.

5.a. This may include assessment information, medical history, strengths, weakness, and interests.

5.b. Use the resources for #4 here as well to generate ideas. You may also wish to have the events calendar from your newspaper handy for additional assistance. The yellow pages of your local telephone book may also be helpful.

5.c.–d. The previously mentioned resources will be helpful here, too. Additionally, your community may have a specific volunteer agency coordination center for seniors.

Follow-up

Refer to the chart below for the appropriate evaluative source most helpful in assuring that your students integrate the information from this exercise.

Application of Competencies (end of chapter 6 in CCOT)	Performance Skills (end of chapter 6 in CCOT)	Appendix (in CCOT)	Clinical Competency Checklist (appendix in IM)
X			

Intervention Planning

Study Questions–Key Terms/Readings

Use the chart below to find information addressing each study question. Look up the key terms in the sources given in the suggested readings column. Refer to the index, the table of contents (T.O.C.), or other locations as indicated.

Study Questions	Key Terms	Suggested Readings
1.	Treatment planning, factors in	Larson—index
2.	Treatment planing, factors in	Larson—index
3.a.–e.	Treatment plans	Lewis—index
4.	Modalities and Treatment in Occupational Therapy	Lewis—T.O.C.
5.a.	Chronic obstructive pulmonary disease (COPD)	Neidstadt—index
	Chronic obstructive pulmonary disease (COPD)	Lewis—index
b.	Parkinson's disease	Lewis—index
c.	Cancer, treatment for	Neidstadt—index
d.	Diabetes mellitus	Lewis—index
e.	Cerebral vascular accident	Lewis—index
f.	Myocardial infarction; Congestive heart failure	Neidstadt—index
6.a.	Aquatic therapy	Lewis—index
b.	Pet therapy	Lewis—index
c.	Horticulture therapy	Lewis—index
d.	Exercise	Lewis—index
e.	Cooking	Lewis—index
f.	Crafts	Lewis—index
g.	Life review	Lewis—index

Activity–Teaching Strategies

1.a.–b. Use case studies #57, #58, #59, #61, #62, and #63. Vary the cultural backgrounds of the clients. Have flip charts in the room for the students to write completed plans. If time does not allow all groups to share their treatment plans, students may review the information on the flip charts. Make copies of the Intervention Plan so the students may write notes directly on these when other groups are sharing.

Follow-up

Refer to the chart below for the appropriate evaluative source most helpful in assuring that your students integrate the information from this exercise.

Application of Competencies (end of chapter 6 in CCOT)	Performance Skills (end of chapter 6 in CCOT)	Appendix (in CCOT)	Clinical Competency Checklist (appendix in IM)
X	6A, 6E		X

Reminiscence and Life Review

Study Questions–Key Terms/Readings

Use the chart below to find information addressing each study question. Look up the key terms in the sources given in the suggested readings column. Refer to the index, the table of contents (T.O.C.), or other locations as indicated.

Study Questions	Key Terms	Suggested Readings
1.a.–b.	Life review; Reminiscence	Lewis—index
c.	Life stories	Larson—index
2.	Life review; Reminiscence	Lewis—index
3.	Life review; Reminiscence	Lewis—index
4.	Life review; Reminiscence	Lewis—index
5.	Life review; Reminiscence	Lewis—index
6.	A Developmental Approach	Cole—T.O.C.
7.	A Developmental Approach	Cole—T.O.C.
8.	Life review; Reminiscence	Lewis—index

Activity–Teaching Strategies

1. Your goal is to have the students share memories, learn more about each other, and demonstrate how enjoyable reminiscing can be. In lieu of the suggested games, make up your own reminiscing activity. Generate questions that most of the students can relate to about their past. Questions about things that promote sharing make for a lively discussion, for example, a school dance, when they learned there was no Santa Claus, or getting their driver's license.

2.a. You will want your students to experience reminiscing firsthand so they can begin to understand the full therapeutic benefit of this intervention. Begin this activity in class to assist the students in getting organized. Time outside of class may be needed for students to finish preparation. Have the groups sign up for a theme for their reminiscing/life review group so that each group will present a different theme. The students may repeat this activity in an environment for the elderly as a service learning project.

2.b. Organize groups according to students needs, for example, divide cliques of students or pair differently-abled students together.

2.c. Use a more formal leadership critique format as found in Cole (1998).

Follow-up

Refer to the chart below for the appropriate evaluative source most helpful in assuring that your students integrate the information from this exercise.

Application of Competencies (end of chapter 6 in CCOT)	Performance Skills (end of chapter 6 in CCOT)	Appendix (in CCOT)	Clinical Competency Checklist (appendix in IM)
X	6B	B: Therapeutic Use of Self-Anlaysis	X

Terminal Illness

Study Questions–Key Terms/Readings

Use the chart below to find information addressing each study question. Look up the key terms in the sources given in the suggested readings column. Refer to the index, the table of contents (T.O.C.), or other locations as indicated.

Study Questions	Key Terms	Suggested Readings
1.	Kubler-Ross, E.	Lewis—index
2.a.–b.	Death, Dying, Bereavement, and Grief: Treatment of the Terminally Ill Elderly	Lewis—T.O.C.
3.	Death, Dying, Bereavement, and Grief: Treatment of the Terminally Ill Elderly	Lewis—T.O.C.
4.	Death, Dying, Bereavement, and Grief: Treatment of the Terminally Ill Elderly	Lewis—T.O.C.
5.	Occupational Therapy and Hospice	AOTA(1998)—T.O.C.
6.	Providing Services for Persons with HIV/AIDS and Their Caregivers	AOTA(1998)—T.O.C.
7.	Reflective	
8.	Caregivers, death and dying responses	Davis—index
9.	Communicating with the Dying and Their Families	Davis—T.O.C.
10.	Reflective	

Activity–Teaching Strategies

1. Set the tone for confidentiality and honesty for sharing within the class. To encourage sharing you may wish to answer the study questions yourself and share some of your thoughts. Smaller groups tend to facilitate more extensive sharing.

2. Use case studies #55 and #64. Use a video on death and dying as an additional activity to get in touch with the person experiencing the dying process.

3. It is important to let the students know that they cannot avoid the issue of death in any area of practice. By facing and dealing with their personal feelings regarding life and death as well as by working with the terminally ill, they will be better prepared to work with their future clients.

Follow-up

Refer to the chart below for the appropriate evaluative source most helpful in assuring that your students integrate the information from this exercise.

Application of Competencies (end of chapter 6 in CCOT)	Performance Skills (end of chapter 6 in CCOT)	Appendix (in CCOT)	Clinical Competency Checklist (appendix in IM)
X			

Activity Programming

Study Questions–Key Terms/Readings

Use the chart below to find information addressing each study question. Look up the key terms in the sources given in the suggested readings column. Refer to the index, the table of contents (T.O.C.), or other locations as indicated.

Study Questions	Key Terms	Suggested Readings
1.	Activity programming, role of an activity professional	Miller—index
2.	Purpose of activities	Miller—index
3.	Needs of residents in long term care; Purpose of activities	Miller—index
4.	Qualifications of activity professionals, nursing, and skilled nursing facilities	Miller—index
5.	The Assessment Process	Miller—T.O.C.
6.	Precautions, potential precautions, precautions list	Miller—index
7.a.–k.	Scope of program; Modes of service delivery	Miller—index
8.	The Activity Director and Professionalism	Miller—T.O.C.
	Professional credentials	Neidstadt—index
	Roles and Function Papers: Occupational Therapy Roles	AOTA(latest edition)—T.O.C.

Activity–Teaching Strategies

1.a. Use activity calendars from various facilities for comparison. Determine the characteristics that are involved in each activity considering only those prominent characteristics that are most used, not necessarily every one that may be involved.

1.b. Comparing activity programs will be interesting. With their OT background, students should quickly be able to identify areas not addressed by a particular facility's program. Discuss any regulations that may apply to activity directors in your state (e.g., Title 22 in California).

1.c.–d. Making an actual calendar helps students try on the role of activities professional. This job option will be more viable in some areas of the country than in others.

1.e. All ideas can be merged into one calendar or ideas can be shared among the group, generating numerous "revised" calendars.

Follow-up

Refer to the chart below for the appropriate evaluative source most helpful in assuring that your students integrate the information from this exercise.

Application of Competencies (end of chapter 6 in CCOT)	Performance Skills (end of chapter 6 in CCOT)	Appendix (in CCOT)	Clinical Competency Checklist (appendix in IM)
X			

Section 6

Performance Skill 6A — Adding to Your File

Add to the list of targeted areas as appropriate for your students. Require students to select activities that can be purchased economically. This restriction gives them experience with real life as budgets may be reduced in long-term care settings. Assign students to select activities for a specific practice setting such as home health or a skilled nursing facility.

Performance Skill 6B — Present a Reminiscing Activity

Use this activity as an opportunity for the students to see how much socialization can be prompted by leading a reminiscing group. If you have students plan this activity for an actual group in a skilled nursing facility or retirement home, have them also plan the needed adaptations the group members may need.

Performance Skill 6C — Prepare/Present a Group Activity

Arrange for students to present their groups at a local nursing home or retirement community. Alternatively, have students initiate their own contacts in the community. If groups are presented simultaneously, organize the location so that you can move easily from group to group to evaluate their performances and be available to answer questions and assist as needed. If possible, have students visit the actual site as part of the planning process. This preliminary visit will help them to know what to expect so they can plan activities accordingly. Have students orally review their plans with you so that you can provide assistance in making sure their plans are in alignment with the purpose of the group and the functioning level of the clients.

Performance Skill 6D — Health and Wellness Presentation

Have a class representative responsible for contacting a local facility to determine the current needs of the residents. Review the information the students plan to present in order to ensure the accuracy of the information and to facilitate a successful presentation.

Performance Skill 6E — Intervention Planning

For OTA students, provide the initial note and initial goals, having them complete the plan with appropriate activities. Have them revise the goals based on a client's hypothetical progress. Use any of the case studies at the end of this chapter or generate one of your own. Predetermine the practice setting as well as the frequency and duration with which treatment will be provided in order to give the students a greater challenge in planning treatment.

Performance Skill 6F   Home Assessment

Make a drawing of your house to serve as an example for the students. When students make their drawings, if major changes are needed to make their homes accessible (such as adding an elevator or first floor bathroom), have the students determine a rough estimate of the costs needed to complete such additions or modifications. If the students rent or lease their property, have them contact their landlords to see if "hypothetically" their recommended changes could be made. Have students discuss their adaptations with the class.

References

American Occupational Therapy Association. latest edition. *Reference Manual of the Official Documents of the American Occupational Therapy Association.* Bethesda, MD: Author.

American Occupational Therapy Association. 1998. *Reference Manual of the Official Documents of the American Occupational Therapy Association.* Bethesda, MD: Author.

Asher, I. E. 1996. *Occupational Therapy Assessment Tools: An Annotated Index.* 2d ed. Bethesda. MD: American Occupational Therapy Association.

A/V Health Services. n.d. *Adapting the Home for the Physically Challenged.* Roanoke, VA: Author.

Bayles, K. A., and C. K. Tomoeda. 1997. *Pastimes.* San Antonio, TX: Therapy Skill Builders.

Christiansen, C., ed. 2000. *Ways of Living: Self-Care Strategies for Special Needs.* 2d ed. Rockville, MD: American Occupational Therapy Association.

Cole, M. D. 1998. *Group Dynamics in Occupational Therapy: The Theoretical Basis and Practice Application of Group Treatment.* 2d ed. Thorofare, NJ: Slack.

Davis, C. M. 1998. *Patient Practitioner Interaction: An Experiential Manual for Developing the Art of Health Care.* 3d ed. Thorofare, NJ: Slack.

Dempsey-Lyle, S., and T. L. Hoffman. n.d. *Into Aging: Understanding Issues Affecting the Later Stages of Life.* Thorofare, NJ: Slack.

Early, M. B. 1998. *Physical Dysfunction Practice Skills for the Occupational Therapy Assistant.* St. Louis, MO: Mosby.

Emlet, C. A., J. L. Crabtree, V. A. Condon, and L. A. Treml. 1996. *In-Home Assessment of Older Adults: An Interdisciplinary Approach.* Gaithersburg, MD: Aspen Publishers.

Folstein, M. F., S. E. Folstein, and P. R. Mettugn. 1975. "Minimental State: A Practical Method for Grading the Cognitive-State of Patients for the Clinician." *Journal of Psychiatric Research,* 12: 189–198.

Holden, U., and R. T. Woods. 1995. *Positive Approaches to Dementia Care.* 3d ed. Edinburgh: Churchill Livingstone.

Hutchins, B. 1991. *Managing Dysphasia.* Tucson, AZ: Therapy Skill Builders.

Isaacs, B., and A. Kinnie. 1973. The Set Test as an Aid to the Detection of Dementia in Old People. *British Journal of Psychiatry,* 123:467.

Larson, K. A., R. G. Stevens-Ratchford, L. Pedretti, and J. L. Crabtree, eds. 1996. *ROTE: The Role of Occupational Therapy with the Elderly.* Bethesda, MD: American Occupational Therapy Association.

Lewis, S. C. 1989. *Elder Care in Occupational Therapy.* Thorofare, NJ: Slack.

MacLay, E. 1977. *Green Winter: Celebration of Old Age.* New York: Reader's Digest Press.

Melvin, J. L. 1989. *Rheumatic Disease in the Adult and Child: Occupational Therapy and Rehabilitation.* 3d ed. Philadelphia: F. A. Davis.

Michelson, B. 1985. *A Slice of Life.* DeKalb, IL: Author.

MIller, M. E., C. W. Peckham, and A. B. Peckham. 1995. *Activities Keep Me Going and*

Going. Vol. 2. Centerville, OH: Macro Printed Products.

Neidstadt, M. E., and E. B. Crepeau. eds. 1998. *Willard and Spackman's Occupational Therapy.* 9th ed. Philadelphia: Lippincott.

Paracheck, J. F. 1986. *Paracheck Geriatric Rating Scale.* 3d ed. Glendale, AZ: Center for Neurodevelopmental Studies.

Pierson, F. M. 1999. *Principles and Techniques of Patient Care.* 2d ed. Philadelphia: W. B. Saunders.

Platt, J. V., R. Begun, and E. D. Murphy. 1992a. *Daily Activities After Your Total Hip Replacement.* Bethesda, MD: American Occupational Therapy Association.

Platt, J. V., R. Begun, and E. D. Murphy. 1992b. *Daily Activities After Your Total Knee Replacement.* Bethesda, MD: American Occupational Therapy Association.

Reed, K. L. 1991. *Quick Reference to Occupational Therapy.* Gaithersburg, MD: Aspen Publishers.

Ross, M. 1997. *Integrative Group Therapy: Mobilizing Coping Abilities with the Five-Stage Group.* Bethesda, MD: American Occupational Therapy Association.

Seaver, A. M. H. 1994. "My World Now." In *The Blair Reader.* L. G. Kriszner and S. R. Mandell. eds. Upper Saddle River, NJ: Prentice Hall.

St. Mary's Hospital Medical Center and the Board of Regents of the University of Wisconsin System. 1984. *ROM Dance.* Madison, WI: WHA Television and St. Mary's Hospital Medical Center in Madison.

Watts, J. H., C. Brollier, D. F. Bauer, and W. Schmidt. 1989. The Assessment of Occupational Therapy Functioning. 2d ed. In *Instrument Development in Occupational Therapy.* J. H. Watts and C. Brollier. eds. New York: Haworth.

Appendix
Clinical Competency Checklist

Clinical Competency Checklist A: Skill Assessment (Self/Instructor/Other) and
Clinical Competency Checklist B: Skill Assessment (Summary):

The list of italicized tasks in these charts have been compiled from the Performance Skills at the end of each chapter that students were directed to complete in the CCOT. The list of nonitalicized tasks in these charts have been compiled from tasks within each chapter that students have been directed to complete during the activity portion of each exercise. Complete Checklist A: Skill Assessment (Self/Instructor/Other) on students as they progress through the completion of each task. Alternatively, or in addition, have the student's clinical supervisor(s) complete this checklist. Direct the student to do the same critiquing his or her own performance. Make as many copies of this form as needed.

Upon completion of Clinical Competency Checklist A: Skill Assessment (Self/Instructor/Other), have students summarize the data from all reviewers of their performance onto the Clinical Competency Checklist B: Skill Assessment (Summary). Have the students include the critique of their performance and plan for improvement in their portfolio. This would be a way of showing growth and evidence of continued learning.

Clinical Competency Checklist C: Professional Behavior Assessment (Self/Peer/Instructor/Other) and
Clinical Competency Checklist D: Professional Behavior Assessment (Summary):

The lists of performance behaviors in these checklists are those important for professional practice in the health care field. Such behaviors will affect a student's job performance and ability to deliver effective health care services. Have the Clinical Competency Checklist C: Professional Behavior Assessment (Self/Peer/Instructor/Other) completed by the student and/or his/her instructors, peers, and clinical supervisor(s), making as many copies of this form as needed. Completion of this form can occur at any time during the student's educational experience such as following the completion of group projects, at the end of a grading period, or at the end of a fieldwork experience.

Upon completion of the Clinical Competency Checklist C: Professional Behavior Assessment (Self/Peer/Instructor/Other), have students summarize the data from all the reviewers of their behavior onto the Clinical Competency Checklist D: Professional Behavior Assessment (Summary). Have the students include the critique of their performance and plan for improvement in their portfolio. This would be another way of showing growth and evidence of continued learning.

Clinical Competency Checklist
A: Skill Assessment
(Self/Instructor/Other)

Name:_____   Date:_____

Legend
Exemplary: Able to teach others **Mastered:** Meets requirements **Needs Improvement:** Unable to demonstrate skill consistently

Using the legend above, initial the following boxes and fill in the date the individual named above completed the following tasks. Compile this information on the Clinical Competency Checklist B: Skill Assessment (Summary).

Chapter one

	Exemplary	Mastered	Needs Improvement	Comments
Craft Completion				
Occupational Analysis				
Adapting an Occupation				
Developing Your File				
Cultural Explanation				

Chapter Two

Teaching an Occupation				
Leading a Group				
Public Relations/Service Learning				
Therapeutic Use of Self				
Mock Interview				

Chapter Three

Adding to Your Files				
Toy Adaptation				
Adaptive Equipment Construction				
Standardized Testing				
Intervention Planning				
Document observations				

	Exemplary	Mastered	Needs Improvement	Comments
Performed various standardized assessments				
Performed passive range of motion				
Utilized proper body mechanics				
Performed lifting techniques for child				
Performed lifting techniques with assist				
Utilized positioning equipment				
Demonstrated handling techniques for feeding				
Demonstrated oral motor techniques				
Analyzed handwriting				
Constructed switch				
Constructed triwall equipment				

Chapter Four

	Exemplary	Mastered	Needs Improvement	Comments
Adding to Your Files				
Interview				
Planning a Group				
Group Activity				
Teaching a Basic Life Task				
More Practice with Your Teaching				
Intervention Planning				
Performed standardized testing				
Led a group				
Redirected inappropriate behavior				

Chapter Five

	Exemplary	Mastered	Needs Improvement	Comments
Disability Simulation				
Fabrication of Adaptive Device				
Adding to Your Files				
Activity Adaptation				

	Exemplary	Mastered	Needs Improvement	Comments
Intervention Planning				
Nontraditional Intervention				
Performed Range of Motion Check				
Demonstrated body mechanics				
Performed standing transfers				
Performed sliding board transfers				
Moved and positioned client in bed				
Measured range of motion				
Performed passive range of motion				
Positioned client in bed				
Applied basic NDT techniques				
Applied basic PNF techniques				
Taught one-handed dressing				
Taught spinal cord dressing				
Selected and used adaptive equipment				
Planned and graded activities of daily living				
Measured strength using dynamometer				
Measured strength using pinch meter				
Performed manual muscle testing				
Completed basic wheelchair measuring and fitting				
Taught wheelchair maneuverability				
Taught wheelchair maintenance				
Tested sensation				
Utilized homemaking in treatment				

	Exemplary	Mastered	Needs Improvement	Comments
Selected therapeutic occupations				
Fabricated static hand splints				
Demonstrated computer skills for patient treatment				
Administered standardized tests				
Performed vital signs				

Chapter Six

	Exemplary	Mastered	Needs Improvement	Comments
Adding to Your Files				
Present a Reminiscing Activity				
Prepare/Present Group				
Health and Wellness Presentation				
Intervention Planning				
Home Assessment				
Performed standardized tests				
Conducted interview				

Clinical Competency Checklist
B: Skill Assessment (Summary)

Name:_____   Date:_____

Legend
Exemplary: Able to teach others **Mastered:** Meets requirements **Needs Improvement:** Unable to demonstrate skill consistently

1. Compile this summary after receiving feedback on the Clinical Competency Checklist A: Skill Assessment (Self/Instructor/Other). Total the responses from the individuals who completed that checklist for you and note them in the corresponding boxes below. Use this summary data to critique your strengths and areas of concern in order to make a plan that will improve your competence as a future practitioner and team member.

Chapter one	Exemplary	Mastered	Needs Improvement	Comments
Craft Completion				
Occupational Analysis				
Adapting an Occupation				
Developing Your File				
Cultural Explanation				
Chapter Two				
Teaching an Occupation				
Leading a Group				
Public Relations/Service Learning				
Therapeutic Use of Self				
Mock Interview				
Chapter Three				
Adding to Your Files				
Toy Adaptation				
Adaptive Equipment Construction				
Standardized Testing				
Intervention Planning				
Documentation of observations				

	Exemplary	Mastered	Needs Improvement	Comments
Performed various standardized assessments				
Performed passive range of motion				
Utilized proper body mechanics				
Performed lifting techniques for child				
Performed lifting techniques with assist				
Utilized positioning equipment				
Demonstrated handling techniques for feeding				
Demonstrated oral motor techniques				
Analyzed handwriting				
Constructed switch				
Constructed triwall equipment				

Chapter Four

	Exemplary	Mastered	Needs Improvement	Comments
Adding to Your Files				
Interview				
Planning a Group				
Group Activity				
Teaching a Basic Life Task				
More Practice with Your Teaching				
Intervention Planning				
Performed standardized testing				
Group Leadership skills				
Ability to redirect inappropriate behavior				

Chapter Five

	Exemplary	Mastered	Needs Improvement	Comments
Disability Simulation				
Fabrication of Adaptive Device				
Adding to Your Files				
Activity Adaptation				

	Exemplary	Mastered	Needs Improvement	Comments
Intervention Planning				
Nontraditional Intervention				
Proficient in Range of Motion Check				
Correct body mechanics demonstrated				
Performed standing transfers				
Performed sliding board transfers				
Moved and positioned client in bed				
Measured range of motion				
Performed passive range of motion				
Positioned client in bed				
Applied basic NDT techniques				
Applied basic PNF techniques				
Taught one-handed dressing				
Taught spinal cord dressing				
Selected and used adaptive equipment				
Planned and graded activities of daily living				
Measured strength using dynamometer				
Measured strength using pinch meter				
Performed manual muscle testing				
Completed basic wheelchair measuring and fitting				
Taught wheelchair maneuverability				
Taught wheelchair maintenance				
Tested sensation				
Utilized homemaking in treatment				

	Exemplary	Mastered	Needs Improvement	Comments
Selected therapeutic occupations				
Fabricated static hand splints				
Demonstrated computer skills for patient treatment				
Administered standardized tests				
Performed vital signs				

Chapter Six

	Exemplary	Mastered	Needs Improvement	Comments
Adding to Your Files				
Present a Reminiscing Activity				
Prepare/Present Group				
Health and Wellness Presentation				
Intervention Planning				
Home Assessment				
Performed standardized tests				
Interview skills				

2. Critique how your assessment of yourself was similar to and/or different from other's evaluation of your performance.

Similarities	Differences

3. List the items that have consistently been a strength for you.

4. List the items that have consistently been an area of concern for you

5. List the tasks that you have shown improvement in since previous assessments.

6. To what do you attribute these improvements?

7. List the areas of concern and note strategies that will improve your performance. If you are uncertain about how to improve these skills seek the advice of an instructor or advisor.

Areas of concern	Goals	Plan

8. Once completed add this Clinical Competency Checklist, critique, and plan to your portfolio.

Clinical Competency Checklist
C: Professional Behavior Assessment
(Self/Peer/ Instructor/Other)

Name:_____   Date:_____

Legend			
Exemplary Performance	**Consistently done**	**Inconsistently done**	**Inadequate performance**
1	2	3	4

Using the legend above, initial the following boxes according to the performance of the individual named above. Compile this information on the Clinical Competency Checklist D: Professional Behavior Assessment (Summary).

Performance	1	2	3	4	Comments
Appearance					
Attendance					
Communication skills					
Ability to get along with others					
Attitude					
Cooperation					
Dependability					
Honesty/integrity					
Initiation /motivation					
Organizational ability					
Problem-solving					
Punctuality					
Self-control					
Work ethic					
Knowledgeable of OT information					
Assertive behavior					
Attention to task					
Ability to give feedback					
Ability to receive feedback					
Written communication skills					
Ability to identify strengths and concerns in self					
Ability to listen to others					

Completed by:

Recommendations:

Clinical Competency Checklist
D: Professional Behavior Assessment (Summary)

Name:_____   Date:_____

1. Complete this summary checklist after receiving the feedback from the Clinical Competency Checklist C: Professional Behavior Assessment (Self/Peer/Instructor/Other) completed by your peers, instructors, and others. Total the responses and from those individuals and note them in the corresponding boxes below. Use this summary data to critique your strengths and areas of concern in order to make a plan that will improve your competence as a future practitioner and team member.

Legend			
Exemplary Performance	Consistently done	Inconsistently done	Inadequate performance
1	2	3	4

Performance	1	2	3	4	Comments
Appearance					
Attendance					
Communication skills					
Ability to get along with others					
Attitude					
Cooperation					
Dependability					
Honesty/integrity					
Initiation /motivation					
Organizational ability					
Problem-solving					
Punctuality					
Self-control					
Work ethic					
Knowledgeable of OT information					
Assertive behavior					
Attention to task					
Ability to give feedback					
Ability to receive feedback					

Performance	1	2	3	4	Comments
Written communication skills					
Ability to identify strengths and concerns					
in self					
Ability to listen to others					

2. Critique how your assessment of yourself was similar to and/or different from other's evaluation of your performance.

Similarities	Differences

3. List the items that have consistently been a strength for you.

4. List the items that have consistently been an area of concern for you

5. List the tasks that you have shown improvement in since previous assessments.

6. To what do you attribute these improvements?

7. List the areas of concern and note strategies that will improve your performance. If you are uncertain about how to improve these skills seek the advice of an instructor or advisor.

Areas of concern	Goals	Plan

8. Once completed add this Clinical Competency Checklist, critique, and plan to your portfolio.

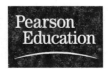

Prentice Hall
Upper Saddle River, NJ 07458
http://www.prenhall.com/health

ISBN 0-8385-1556-8

90000

9 780838 515563